PENGUIN BOOKS

WHAT EVERY PREGNANT WOMAN SHOULD KNOW

Gail Sforza Brewer attended Wells College and holds B.S. and M.A. degrees in communication from Syracuse University and the University of Wisconsin. Mother of three, she has worked as a journalist, college professor, and childbirth educator. She is currently director of instructor training and certification for the Metropolitan New York Childbirth Education Association and teaches childbirth classes in Westchester County, New York.

Tom Brewer, M.D., graduated from Tulane University School of Medicine and completed residency programs in general practice and obstetrics-gynecology. A former research fellow at Howard Hughes Medical Institute in Miami, Florida, and instructor in the Department of Obstetrics-Gynecology at the University of California Medical School, San Francisco, he conducted a demonstration nutrition-education project in the public prenatal clinics of the Contra Costa County, California, Medical Services from 1963 to 1976. His clinical handbook for the practicing physician, *Metabolic Toxemia of Late Pregnancy: A Disease of Malnutrition*, was published in 1966. Dr. Brewer is president of the Society for the Protection of the Unborn through Nutrition (SPUN), a nonprofit organization committed to the establishment of scientific standards of nutrition management in American obstetrics.

WHAT EVERY PREGNANT WOMAN SHOULD KNOW

The Truth about
Diets and Drugs
in Pregnancy

**GAIL SFORZA BREWER
with TOM BREWER, M.D.,
Medical Consultant**

PENGUIN BOOKS

Penguin Books Ltd, Harmondsworth,
Middlesex, England
Penguin Books, 625 Madison Avenue,
New York, New York 10022, U.S.A.
Penguin Books Australia Ltd, Ringwood,
Victoria, Australia
Penguin Books Canada Limited, 2801 John Street,
Markham, Ontario, Canada L3R 1B4
Penguin Books (N.Z.) Ltd, 182–190 Wairau Road,
Auckland 10, New Zealand

First published in the United States of America by
Random House, Inc., 1977
First published in Canada by
Random House of Canada Limited 1977
Published in Penguin Books 1979
Reprinted 1980 (twice), 1981

Library of Congress Cataloging in Publication Data
Brewer, Gail Sforza.
  What every pregnant woman should know.
  Bibliography: p. 231.
  Includes index.
  1. Pregnancy—Nutritional aspects. 2. Fetus,
effect of drugs on the. I. Brewer, Thomas H., joint
author. II. Title.
RG559.B73   1979   618.2'4   79–10441
ISBN 0 14 00.5224 0

Printed in the United States of America by
Offset Paperback Mfrs., Inc., Dallas, Pennsylvania
Set in Times Roman

FOR ALL OUR CHILDREN

Science should always explain obscurity and complexity by clearer and simpler ideas.

—CLAUDE BERNARD, 1865

Nutrition is the most important of all environmental factors in childbearing whether the problem is considered from the point of view of the mother or that of the offspring.

—SIR EDWARD MELLANBY, 1933

ACKNOWLEDGMENTS

A special note of thanks to several people whose interest and enthusiasm helped make this book possible:

to Jay Hodin, Executive Director of SPUN (the Society for the Protection of the Unborn through Nutrition), for allowing access to unpublished materials on malnutrition and developmental disabilities;

to Judy Norsigian of the Boston Women's Health Book Collective for assistance in finding the right publisher;

to Ann Anderson, Linda Chastain, Susan Dart, Nancy Gotsch, Elsie Sforza and Mary Wilkinson for sharing some of their favorite family recipes;

to Robert Mendelsohn, M.D., Douglas Shanklin, M.D., Mary Jane Gray, M.D., and Harold Schulman, M.D., for reviewing the manuscript before publication;

and to Charlotte Mayerson, the editor who provided invaluable perspective and guidance from the outset of this project. Without her initial perceptions of the direction the book should take, it could never have appeared in this form.

Croton-on-Hudson, New York
March 8, 1977

CONTENTS

WHAT EVERY
PREGNANT
WOMAN
SHOULD
KNOW

A ROUTINE OFFICE VISIT

"Let's step up on the scales first," the nurse directed.

Eve Gilbert had been preparing for this moment for two days —eating little and, last night, taking a laxative, anticipating the big brunch she planned to share with her husband, Dick, after her appointment. Though it was the middle of January, she wore a sleeveless summer dress and no underwear, hoping to save a few extra ounces from being permanently entered on her chart in the column marked "Weight."

"One forty-six," the nurse intoned. "You've gained six pounds this month. That makes twenty-four altogether. Doctor won't be too happy about this. You're the third one this morning. Must be the holidays! You'll regret all that turkey and eggnog next summer on the beach, I can tell you that! And all that weight won't do the baby any good, either. What kid wants a fat mother?" Shaking her head, she wrote "146" on the chart, set Eve up on the examining table, then swept out. The nurse knew how Dr. Finley felt about women gaining too much weight, so she took special care to give each one advice about dieting right after the "weigh-in." It was one of the most important parts of her job.

Eve wished Dick had come with her. Last month she had gained five pounds. Dr. Finley had said then that she had only six pounds to go, and it was up to her how long she took to gain them. Now, with the birth of her baby still eight weeks away, she had reached the limit.

The nurse's remark about too much weight harming the baby worried her. Yet, Eve was hungry much of the time. She felt tired and irritable when she didn't eat. She wondered if this was normal in pregnancy. Two of her friends had gone to Dr. Finley and he had given them diet pills to control their appetites. Now, after their babies were born, they looked so trim. It was hard to tell they had ever had a baby and they credited Dr. Finley's careful watch on their weight for their good figures.

Eve decided to ask the doctor to help her, too, since she was having so much trouble doing it on her own. She wrote "Pills?" at the bottom of her list of questions for the day, hoping he would have time to talk. She always felt guilty about taking too much time in the office, even when she had important questions.

"Good morning, Eve," Dr. Finley boomed. She liked his friendly manner, which added to her confidence in him. "How are you and junior doing today?" He strode directly to the desk where the nurse had arranged Eve's file, glanced at the column marked "Weight" and turned to her with a more sober expression. "Six pounds, I see. What am I going to do with you gals? Too many holiday parties?"

"Not really, Dr. Finley," Eve started to explain. "I guess I need help to stop eating so much. I've really tried the past few days, but I'm always hungry."

"Well, we can talk about that in a few minutes," he replied. "There are a few other things I want to check first, so we know where we stand."

"Is there something wrong?" she wanted to know.

"Now I didn't say that, did I?"

The nurse brought in the tray with the equipment needed for Eve's examination: fetoscope, tape measure, blood pressure apparatus and thermometer. The last she placed under Eve's tongue while Dr. Finley took Eve's pulse. Then he attached the blood pressure cuff above Eve's elbow, pumped it up, released the pressure, said "Hmm," then repeated the procedure. The nurse stood ready by the desk to fill in the numbers on Eve's chart. Eve stared at the ceiling with the thermometer under her tongue, pretending not to listen to them as they assigned numerical values to her body's functions.

"One thirty over eighty," Finley reported.

"One thirty over eighty," the nurse wrote.

"Pulse seventy-six."

"Seventy-six."

Placing the fetoscope on her abdomen, the doctor listened for the familiar thumping of a healthy baby's heart. After fifteen seconds he announced, "One forty."

Next he stretched the tape measure from Eve's pubic bone up over her protruding tummy to the topmost margin of her growing uterus. "Twenty-six c-m's," he relayed.

Finally, with both hands he pressed on Eve's middle in several places, chuckled when the baby kicked, then stood back and said, "The baby's in good position, head down, so you're both in fine shape. After you're back together I'll give you a little stick in the finger to check your blood count."

The sample of blood was analyzed by the office technician. It was the last number to be entered on Eve's chart for the day; her urine test was normal. The nurse poked her head through the doorway en route to her next "weigh-in."

"Hematocrit thirty-seven," she said. "Urine negative."

"Is that okay?" Eve asked, knowing she hadn't had a blood test since her first appointment months ago.

"Just fine," Dr. Finley answered. "Are you taking the vitamins and iron pills I prescribed for you?"

"Yes, of course," Eve replied.

"Then we won't have any problems with anemia, will we?" Finley smiled.

"Now," the doctor began as he closed the file and looked at her face for the first time that morning, "any questions?"

Yes, there were advantages and disadvantages to both formula and breast-feeding. The nurse could give her a pamphlet about infant feeding on the way out. Each mother must decide which type of feeding suited her best.

Yes, the hospital did allow fathers to participate in the birth and help in the care of their newborn babies, if the mother had a private room. The nurse could arrange a private room if Eve decided she wanted to have the baby with her, but many of his patients had complained about being tired after having "rooming-in."

Yes, it would be all right for her to continue her weekly swim at the Y, as long as she didn't overexert herself. Walking was also good exercise, he thought, and a good way to prevent leg cramps.

"Pills?" was the last entry on her list.

She summoned her courage.

"Dr. Finley, what can I do about my weight? I know I've already gained the twenty-four pounds you said were okay. What should I eat? Can you give me some diet pills so I don't feel so hungry?" Eve asked nervously.

"That's what I wanted to discuss, too, Eve," he said seriously. "I used to give diet pills, but some recent studies have shown that they don't work to reduce weight permanently and that they may have some bad effects on the baby. Just to be safe, we should try another approach for the next few weeks and see how it works."

He reached into a file cabinet next to the desk and pulled out a sheet of paper which he handed to Eve.

"This is a low-calorie, low-salt diet plan for pregnancy. We use this now instead of diet pills. It tells you just which foods to eat and which to avoid. You see, we can't tell just by looking, but it may be that some of the weight you've put on already is just water your body is retaining. Salt does that, you know. So, if you cut down on your salt and cut back on your calories, we should see some loss of weight in a week or two. Have you noticed any swelling in your feet and ankles?"

Eve nodded, "Just toward the end of the day a little bit. Is it dangerous?"

"No. Swelling of the ankles is pretty common. The weight of the baby pressing down on veins in the pelvis usually causes it. But," and he paused for emphasis, "if you notice any swelling of your face, or your rings get tight, that would be a sign of toxemia. You'd call me right away, agreed?"

She murmured assent, busily examining the lists of permitted and not-permitted foods, thinking she'd have to forget the brunch with Dick. She'd just sip some orange juice while he ate.

The doctor was on his way out the door.

Eve looked up gratefully. "Thank you, Dr. Finley. I'll do everything the diet sheet says. I'm sorry to have taken so much of your time today."

2
THE QUESTION
DOCTORS DON'T ASK

There are three million Eves and over twenty thousand Dr. Finleys re-enacting the preceding scene each year in the United States.

On the surface it appears to be a well-conducted, even amiable interchange—the sort many women can remember as part of their pregnancy experience. A closer look reveals a grave omission which jeopardizes every pregnant woman and every unborn baby. This omission occurs routinely because the standards which determine the type of prenatal care given to pregnant women in America are deficient. They do not require that doctors ask each mother one simple, potentially lifesaving question:

"What have you been eating?"

Until sound nutrition is accorded first priority in American obstetrical practice, all mothers must be considered "high-risk," endangered by the common pregnancy complications now known to be nutritional in origin.

The lack of attention given to pregnant women's nutrition in our country contributes heavily to some disturbing facts of contemporary life: the United States lags far behind many other advanced countries in terms of the health of our mothers and babies. Out of every thousand born, we lose eighteen babies in the first year of life, placing us sixteenth in the world according to international statistics compiled by the United Nations.

The incidence of low-birth-weight babies (under five and a half pounds at birth) born to mothers in all economic groups has risen sharply since 1960. Birth weight is the most important factor in predicting a child's future health and mental development. The correlation between low birth weight and a wide range of developmental disorders is highly significant and alarming. This sudden rise in low-birth-weight babies has not occurred in other industrialized countries which report lower infant mortality statistics.

There has been an upsurge in the number of brain-damaged, hyperkinetic and learning-disabled children entering our nation's schools since the early 1960's. This has happened at a time when birth rates have been declining. Formerly considered a problem largely of inner-city schools, the number of these children has reached epidemic proportions in even the most affluent areas. For example, officials in Monroe County, New York, a suburb of Rochester, report that 25 percent of their students are affected.

For the past forty years research has been conducted all over the world which concretely links maternal malnutrition with a host of obstetric and pediatric complications. Yet in 1975 the U.S. Department of Health, Education and Welfare published research which concluded that the total number of pregnant women suffering from malnutrition—serious enough to endanger their babies—was more than 945,000. Roughly one in three pregnant women in America falls into the malnourished group!

It is our opinion, based on analysis of this research and Tom's own work with pregnant women, that much of the pregnancy malnutrition found in the United States is attributable to unscientific methods of nutrition management which have become entrenched in American obstetrics. Our physicians, almost without exception, have been trained to demand compliance with weight control regimens in pregnancy, irrespective of the mother's nutritional needs. Most of these programs feature low-calorie, low-salt diets and the use of salt diuretics (water pills). They take into account neither the serious medical consequences of such dietary practices nor what is known about human nutrition.

As it stands now, most doctors have never taken a course in applied human nutrition. No medical school in the United States requires such a course of its students. As Dr. Frederick Zuspan, editor of *The American Journal of Obstetrics and Gynecology*, commented in August, 1976:

> Most medical students, interns, and practicing physicians do not know or appreciate good nutrition. This change must begin in the medical schools.

Doctors currently in training need to learn about the protective benefits of sound pregnancy nutrition. Just as important, doctors already practicing must also be educated and begin to apply the scientific research in nutrition to routine prenatal care.

In this they have much to learn from ranchers, farmers and veterinarians who are taught the importance of feeding pregnant animals scientifically. They know exactly what constitutes a healthful diet for a pregnant cow, sheep or horse. And they enthusiastically put into practice what they know. They have to. Some cows are worth $5,000 apiece!

Is a pregnant woman as valuable as a cow? If so, the answer to improving pregnancy outcomes in our country lies in raising the awareness of doctors and women alike to the importance of good nutrition in pregnancy. The idea that pregnancy imposes a special nutritional stress on every woman is not commonly held. On the contrary, letters we have received from thousands of women all

over the country indicate that nutritional nonchalance character-
izes much of the dietary advice given by many American obstetricians. A sampling of the most recent letters illustrates the point:

Little Rock, Arkansas

I am three months along and have had one miscarriage: the
doctor told me I could only gain ten pounds. But is that right?
I don't feel right about it.

Worthington, Ohio

Just last night in our childbirth class one "skinny" gal, four
and a half months pregnant, stated her doctor reduced her
diet to 1,000 calories because she gained seven pounds in
seven weeks. This is the only weight she has gained thus far
in her pregnancy.

Los Angeles County, California

Last week one of my students was told by a young doctor
to lose fifteen pounds (she's due in three weeks) and that if
she didn't she'd have to 'go to County to deliver'—a threat
they often use as it has a horrible reputation in obstetrics.
Many gals are scared into dieting in order to save having to
go there. This doctor also told the woman that it didn't really
matter what she ate as the baby took it all from her anyway!

New York City

I'm a public health nurse involved in a prenatal clinic here;
and in spite of the convincing evidence of harm, the clinic
physicians still order low-salt and weight reduction diets.
They get hysterical over a four-pound weight gain in one
month!

Miami, Florida

I have a student due in December who is underweight for
her height. She is going to a private doctor who does not want

her to gain more than eighteen pounds. One month she gained three pounds and he was very upset about it. He told her not to salt her food.

Boston, Massachusetts

I have been a member of the American Dietetic Association since 1956, have a master's degree in nutrition and have worked in two teaching hospitals in New England. I have talked with many women who are afraid to face the physician because they have gained weight. I have attempted to discuss with these women the need for the basic four food groups emphasizing protein, but unless the physician has asked that they talk to me, they usually pay little attention because it has not come from the doctor.

Memphis, Tennessee

I had a first child who was a low-birth-weight, "toxic" baby due to the severe toxemia I developed in my last trimester of pregnancy. My OB doctor restricted me to *clear liquids only* for six weeks and diuretics daily. I have never received a straight answer to my questions about toxemia and its cause.

Ann Arbor, Michigan

When I was pregnant, my doctor told me I had preeclampsia, but did not elaborate to my satisfaction. Although I had regular prenatal checkups, no one even mentioned the possibility of toxemia to me until my blood pressure continued to rise on the delivery table. If I really had toxemia, shouldn't a doctor have known before? Is toxemia just a name that is applied to several symptoms, including weight gain, swelling, headaches, etc? I am especially interested in the relationship of nutrition to toxemia.

Havelock, North Carolina

When I went for my first prenatal, I was told to go on a salt-free diet and to eat sparingly so I would not gain "too much weight." All during my pregnancy my father told me I wasn't eating right, regardless of what the doctors were telling me to eat. I thought he was just being old-fashioned with his views of pregnancy and nutrition.

During the first six months I was always exhausted and developed severe anemia. I also developed severe kidney infections and toxemia. In the beginning of my eighth month, the toxemia was so severe I was hospitalized. I was placed on a diet of 24 ounces of skim milk and 24 ounces of dietetic orange juice daily.

On the third day in the hospital, I went into premature labor and my daughter was born six hours later. She had yellow jaundice, respiratory difficulty and weighed four pounds, ten and a half ounces. For the first week of her life she refused to eat. Two months later she died of what the doctors called Sudden Infant Death Syndrome, or crib death.

Middletown, New Jersey

I argued with my obstetrician through two pregnancies to leave me and my thirty-five-pound gain alone. My babies were eight pounds, six ounces and eight pounds, two ounces —and healthy.

Green Bay, Wisconsin

I am a high school home economics teacher and have five children. None was a defective baby, fortunately, because I *ignored* my doctor's accusations that I was gaining weight at a rate twice too fast. I did not argue, but I knew in my bones that my baby was made out of what I ate. I was sufficiently intimidated not to protest, though.

Each of my children weighed between eight and nine pounds. I was the string bean type—can you imagine what shape they would have been in if I gained only fifteen to twenty pounds!

Now in my classes when I tell my students that in somewhere between thirteen and twenty-two other countries a baby has a better chance to live to see its first birthday than in the United States, the students are shocked.

"How could this be? Why?" they ask.

Isn't it ironic that it has been medical advice that has caused devastating effects on these babies and mothers?

What would it take to redirect the efforts of these doctors away from weight control and onto sound nutrition? To make sure that every mother receives proper instruction about her diet? How much would it cost to insure that Dr. Finley asked Eve that all-important question: What have you been eating?

It requires neither the expenditure of vast sums of federal money nor the establishment of special offices and programs dispensing nutrition information. Quite simply, all that is needed is for every obstetrician to learn and pass on to his patients the basics of pregnancy nutrition and to emphasize this information at each prenatal visit. It would not take any more of the busy physician's time to disseminate correct information than is currently spent hounding women about their weight. And mothers would appreciate the chance to cooperate in a program designed to make pregnancy a healthful time for herself and her unborn baby.

The first step is convincing the doctor that the old methods he was taught in medical school have become obsolete in modern prenatal care.

3
WEIGHT CONTROL:
a hazard in pregnancy

The idea that the weight of a pregnant woman should be controlled has been prevalent in obstetrics for a long time. Too long.

As medical knowledge has advanced, particularly about the way the baby develops in utero, it has become clear that the practice of strict weight control benefits neither mother nor child. The thinking of American obstetricians, however, continues to be conditioned by four theories which have been popular for years:

1. Weight restriction is beneficial to the mother because it makes delivery easier.
2. Weight restriction is beneficial to the mother because it prevents toxemia.
3. Weight restriction does not harm the baby because the baby is a parasite, able to take what it needs from the mother.
4. Weight restriction does not harm the baby because the baby's birth weight is determined by heredity.

1. There is no denying that weight restriction results in smaller babies. Nineteenth-century medical school professors from Brunninghausen in 1803 to Prochownick in 1899 wrote extensively on

the subject. But the idea that a smaller baby necessarily makes for an easier delivery overlooks a critical corollary to weight control —nutritional deprivation. In circumstances where mothers are on deficient diets, the weight control that results in a smaller baby is now known to also result in a uterus that is likely to malfunction during labor. Labor is often prolonged in these cases. Sometimes it stops altogether and the uterus must be artificially stimulated by drugs into further contractions. When this fails, Caesarean section is the only recourse. Dr. Cecil Mary Drillien reported in 1958 in the *Journal of OB/GYN of the British Empire* that more maternal complications are associated with low-birth-weight babies than those of normal weight. Among four hundred low-birth-weight infants studied, 52 percent of mothers experienced complications, whereas only 10 percent of the mothers of babies with normal birth weight experienced complications. These observations have been confirmed by many other researchers. Advocating weight control during pregnancy as a way of making labor easier simply does not correspond with the facts.

2. The notion that a mother who gains too much weight in pregnancy is more liable to develop toxemia arose because of confusion about what causes the disease. The predominant theory for many years was the "utero-placental ischemia theory." Its proponents believed that fatty accumulations around the blood vessels in the pelvis interfered with the flow of blood to the uterus. The placenta supposedly responds to the reduced blood flow by releasing an as yet unidentified "x" substance. The "x" factor, the theory holds, causes blood vessels throughout the body to constrict, raising the mother's blood pressure to dangerous levels. Direct damage to the mother's kidneys, liver, brain and other vital organs are also blamed on this constriction of blood vessels.

Were this theory correct, the obstetrician would certainly be justified in controlling the weight gain of every patient. Toxemia is one of the most dangerous pregnancy complications. However, evidence from investigators around the world, reported since the 1930's, points to an entirely different cause of toxemia—maternal malnutrition during pregnancy. This metabolic theory traces the onset of toxemia to a lack of nutrients essential in pregnancy, chiefly protein. Lack of these nutrients results in a malfunctioning liver. Various compensatory mechanisms throughout the body are called into action when liver function fails. These mechanisms account for the high blood pressure and abnormal swelling that characterize toxemia.

3. The "parasite theory" supports weight control because it contends that the developing baby takes priority for essential nutrients over the mother's own tissues. If any necessary nutrients are missing from the mother's diet, the baby is able to extract whatever it needs directly from the mother's body: protein from her muscles, calcium from her bones, etc. In this way, the theory holds, the baby is guaranteed normal physical and mental development in the womb, no matter how malnourished the mother may be. If the baby is small at birth, no one is to worry. These theorists see the small baby as merely perfection in miniature.

4. Enter the "genetic theory" which maintains that the baby's weight and length at birth are inherited traits. If the parents are tall, the baby will be big; if short, small. This theory has been used as a way of explaining the much higher incidence of low birth weight and brain-damaged children among lower income groups in our country. Epilepsy, for instance, is ten times more common among the poor. If these problems can be traced to genetic inferiority, then there is nothing anyone in authority can do except perhaps build more institutions to care for the retarded. If everything about a baby's development is predetermined by the parents' legacy of chromosomes, there is little that can be done to improve the outcome of pregnancy short of choosing the right

ancestors, as one well-known obstetrician has only half-jokingly suggested.

If either the parasite theory or the genetic theory were valid, neither restricting nor supplementing the diets of pregnant women should have any effect on their babies' birth weights. Yet it has been known since the nineteenth century that weight control results in a smaller baby, and Mrs. Agnes Higgins of the Montreal Diet Dispensary has shown over the past twenty years that improving a mother's diet results in a larger newborn.

The four theories discussed above have influenced the training of most obstetricians in practice today, so that weight control remains a fixture in American obstetrics. Doctors continue to seek a definitive answer to an irrelevant question: How much weight can a pregnant woman gain without placing herself or her baby in jeopardy?

The current "magic number" is 24 pounds, accounted for by a prominent obstetrician in this way:

Fetal tissues (baby)	7½ pounds
Placenta	1
Amniotic fluid	2
Organ growth (uterus)	2
Growth of breasts	1½
Increase in blood	3½
Tissue fluid and stored body fat	6½
Total maternal weight gain:	24 pounds

This table appears to be based on a scientific analysis of the various physiologic changes that occur in normal pregnancy. However, recent research demonstrates that when weight control is not practiced and the mother is encouraged to maintain throughout pregnancy optimal nutrition, including adequate salt intake, she commonly gains ten pounds more than this table indicates. Additional circulating blood, tissue fluid and stored fat comprise these ten pounds. This is not excessive, undesirable weight. Rather, as we shall see, this increase is a proven safeguard for mother and baby that is subverted when weight control is practiced in lieu of scientific nutritional counseling.

A booklet published in 1974 by the American College of Obstetricians and Gynecologists contains a chart which indicates that the twenty-four pounds must be gained according to a set pattern in order to minimize obstetrical risks. Deviations from this pattern are to be interpreted as warning signs. A statement accompanying the chart also explains that twenty-four pounds are not to be gained by every pregnant woman. Those who are overweight at conception should have a smaller weight gain because by the end of pregnancy a mother should weigh no more than twenty-four pounds over her "ideal weight" for her height. The determination of appropriate weight gain in any individual case is left to the discretion of the physician.

This chart first appeared in a medical journal, *Clinical Obstetrics,* in 1953. Since its publication many comprehensive clinical studies have been reported in major journals here and abroad.[1] In fact, some of these studies originally were published in ACOG's own journal. Evidence from these more recent investigations leads to the conclusion that for numerous reasons it is hazardous to rely on weight control as a tool for management of human pregnancy. To the contrary, healthier mothers and babies result when the focus is on nutrition, not pounds.

Hytten and Thomson, British investigators writing on maternal physiologic adjustments in pregnancy in a 1970 publication of

[1] See bibliography: Brewer, Eastman, Hamlin, Iyengar, Lowe, Pasamanick, Pike, Platt and Singer.

the National Academy of Science, were struck not by the supposed predictability of weight gain in normal pregnancy, but by its variability. They present convincing evidence that normal pregnancies can take place within a wide range of weight gain and loss, and that the pattern of weight adjustment is a function of individual metabolism and activity. It is, therefore, not wise to attempt to regulate it.

They note that it was hard to find subjects for their research since many—perhaps most—obstetricians advise patients to eat less than their appetites dictate, thus altering the normal adjustments they wanted to study.

The 746 Scottish women chosen for investigation met all the criteria for normality in pregnancy: they were between the ages of twenty to twenty-nine, at least sixty-three inches tall, in good physical condition and were allowed to eat to appetite. All gave birth to normal, healthy babies between the thirty-ninth and the forty-first week of gestation.

A chart showing the distribution of their weight gains over the last twenty weeks of pregnancy disproves every point advanced in the ACOG weight-control chart. Instead of each mother gaining the same amount of weight per week in the last twenty weeks, some mothers gained virtually nothing while others gained over forty pounds! Neither the total number of pounds gained, nor the pattern in which it was gained had any effect on the outcome of pregnancy. *All mothers and all babies were normal.*

Clearly some factor other than the number of pounds gained was responsible for the normal outcomes of these pregnancies. A look at what the mothers were eating, a variable the study failed to detail, would be more productive in terms of providing practical advice for the physician to pass along to his patients.

Of course, if one looks at all the pregnancies in this study and averages the weight gains an absolute number is reached. However, this statistical approach to the question of what is the correct management of an individual pregnant woman can only lead to difficulties. To establish the average of all weight gains in normal pregnancies as some sort of "ideal" to which every individual case must correspond means that only those mothers for whom the "ideal" is physiologically compatible will be managed properly. All others will be coerced into following a pattern which does not foster their most healthful adjustment to pregnancy! In short, they are placed at higher risk of developing complications.

Babies are also more likely to suffer when the obstetrician's attention is devoted to controlling the mother's weight. Low birth weight commonly results when the mother follows advice to restrict calories and salt and to take diuretics during pregnancy. As was pointed out in 1968 by the *National Institutes of Health Collaborative Study of Cerebral Palsy, "Mental Retardation and Other Neurological and Sensory Disorders of Infancy and Childhood,"* the baby who weighs under five and a half pounds at birth is more apt to be afflicted with such defects as mental retardation, cerebral palsy, epilepsy, hyperactivity, learning disabilities, respiratory distress syndrome (RDS) and sudden infant death syndrome (SIDS).

Most doctors know that in the last two months of pregnancy the baby who is developing normally experiences an unparalleled growth spurt. Many seem not to realize that this critical phase of the baby's development can be seriously disrupted by inadequate maternal nutrition during these last few weeks of gestation. When the physician rigidly enforces a weight gain limit, mothers often reach it just as the baby's growth spurt begins. When a mother starts to cut down on her food and salt intake in order not to exceed her doctor's weight limit, she unknowingly begins to starve her unborn baby. It is tragic that as she earnestly strives to carry out her doctor's orders in the belief she is doing the best for herself and her baby, the mother is actually placing them both in jeopardy.

The work of Dr. John Dobbing—a research professor in the Department of Child Health, University of Manchester Medical School, England—explains how interference with maternal nutrition at the end of pregnancy compromises the growth of the baby's brain in particular. In February of 1976, he concluded in a talk at the Montreal Children's Hospital:

> Even mild degrees of maternal undernutrition in the last few weeks of pregnancy can interfere with the normal growth and development of the human fetal brain.

For many years Dobbing has studied how the brain of the unborn baby develops. Identifying two periods of rapid growth of brain cells—the first at twenty weeks gestation and the second at thirty-six weeks, one month before the baby is born—he believes that the developing brain is most vulnerable to the effects of maternal malnutrition at these times.

Since even "mild degrees of maternal undernutrition" can interfere with the baby's brain growth and development, the doctor must recognize what constitutes such "undernutrition," so it can be prevented in every pregnancy.

A sample day's menu from a typical low-salt, low-calorie diet sheet clearly exemplifies the undernutrition Dobbing warned against. Though apparently supplying an amount of high quality protein adequate for pregnancy (approximately 90 grams) its severe restriction of calories and salt makes it a hazard to mother and baby.

The importance of adequate protein intake during pregnancy was proven by the pioneering work of Bertha S. Burke of Harvard. In the 1940's she found that women whose diets contained 45 grams or less of protein a day suffered the highest incidence of stillbirths, neonatal deaths, congenital defects, premature and low-birth-weight babies.

The late Professor Benjamin S. Platt demonstrated at the London School of Tropical Medicine that these disorders could be produced experimentally in animals by limiting protein. One way to do this is by restricting protein intake directly by not allowing the animals to eat protein-rich foods. Another way is to limit the amount of carbohydrates the animals consume. He found that when the calorie intake provided by fats, sugars and starches is reduced below the body's requirements, dietary protein is burned for energy. During pregnancy this means that only the "leftover" protein will be available for growth of the baby and maintenance of maternal health.

A moderately active woman needs approximately 2,600 calories every day to meet her normal energy requirements in the last three months of pregnancy. If she is carrying twins, the figure is closer to 3,100 calories. On the kind of diet recommended for weight control by most obstetricians, she is only going to get 1,700 calories—a deficit of at least 900.

Platt calculated that a deficit of one-third in needed calories results in *one-half the dietary protein being burned for energy*. So, over half the 90 grams of protein the mother is allowed daily on this diet will not be available for building her baby's body and brain.

In other words, the effect of a "low-calorie, low-salt" diet is to put the mother on a "low-protein" diet—less than 45 grams a day —and right into the severely malnourished group Burke identified in the 1940's as being at higher risk.

The undernutrition caused by protein-calorie deficiency is aggravated by drastic restriction of salt to less than two grams a day. When the mother follows this diet, she and her baby are in trouble.

4

LOW-SALT DIETS:
why they don't work

Every day of her life the expectant mother, like every other man and woman, needs salt. Each of the trillions of cells that make up her body testify to this biological necessity. Like the cells of all species evolved from the sea, hers must be continually bathed in salt water to remain healthy.

Her unborn baby shares this legacy. Afloat in a sac filled with hospitable brine, the baby obtains all the salt it needs from the mother's circulating supply. The only way the essential salt will be in the mother's bloodstream is if she eats it. Salt is a component of many foods, in addition to being readily available in its commonest form, ordinary table salt. The placenta permits the transfer of salt from the mother's bloodstream to the baby's from the earliest weeks of pregnancy until the moment of birth.

Every person has many finely tuned mechanisms which work in the body to preserve the appropriate concentration of salt in and around each cell and in the bloodstream. These mechanisms are inter-related, so that a change in salt metabolism which affects one of them causes adjustments in others. Human salt requirements are widely variable depending on an individual's level of physical activity, state of health or illness, and the external temperature and humidity. There is a great deal of concern today about overconsumption of salt in our country. Studies have shown that excess salt intake from infancy onward may result from the intake of prepared foods and snack foods which contain a great deal of salt, but little else nutritionally, and have come to comprise a large part of the diets of many people. While the concern about over-salting may be legitimate in terms of overall public health, there is one group of people for whom over-salting is not a problem— pregnant women. In fact, pregnancy is one condition in which the body requires *more* salt in order to remain healthy. Numerous changes in the mother's body during pregnancy explain this increased need for salt.

Of first importance is the growth and development of the placenta. This organ, unique to pregnancy, makes possible the exchange of all nutrients and waste products between mother and baby. As the baby grows and requires more nourishment, the placenta increases in size to provide it. If the placenta does not grow well, neither can the baby.

As pregnancy progresses, the placenta needs a great deal more blood flowing through it in order to work efficiently. In normal pregnancy, the mother's blood volume must expand by more than 40 percent to meet this metabolic need. Salt is a chief element in maintaining this dramatically expanded blood volume. One of the properties of salt is that it causes the body to retain fluid which, under normal conditions, is retained in the bloodstream for use in placental perfusion. Salt restriction during pregnancy limits the normal expansion of the blood volume. A blood volume below the level needed to service the growing placenta produces disastrous consequences.

Depending on the degree of salt restriction and subsequent blood volume limitation, the placenta may grow slowly or not at all; develop areas of dead tissue (infarcts) which cannot function;

be unable to accomplish the transfer of all needed nutrients to the baby; or even begin to separate from the wall of the uterus, causing hemorrhage and cutting off the baby's oxygen supply. Obviously, when the ability of the placenta to function is impaired, the baby's growth, development and even life are imperiled.

Clinical evidence for this view of the importance of salt in pregnancy was provided in 1958 by Dr. Margaret Robinson, a London obstetrician. Working in a public clinic, she conducted a study of 2,019 pregnant women, chosen at random. Half were instructed to reduce their salt intake; half to increase it. Information about which foods contain high amounts of salt was given to the mothers in the low-salt group. Dr. Robinson did nothing else by way of dietary counseling to influence what the mothers ate. She only asked them to report the amounts of salt they were eating.

Unfortunately, not all the high-salt foods on the restricted list are nutritionally deficient. For instance, many, like milk, eggs, salty cheeses, salty fish and salty meat products are important sources of essential high-quality proteins. Since this study was conducted with low-income mothers for the most part, the effect of banning these foods from the diet because of their salt content was also to ban the lower-priced sources of excellent protein. Consequently, when the mothers followed the diet and were unable to afford higher-priced protein foods, such as lean meat, they were not only on a low-salt diet but on a low-protein one as well. So, the outcome of this study is due not merely to salt-restriction alone, but to a combination of salt and protein restriction. Since imposition of a low-salt regimen on a pregnant mother may well mean protein deprivation as well, the results of Robinson's work are very significant:

The low-salt group had nearly three times more damaged placentas, two and a half times more toxemia and twice the number of infant deaths.

The high-salt group fared better in other ways. They had fewer delivery complications and even a reduced incidence of leg cramps during pregnancy than mothers in the low-salt group.

The inescapable conclusion is that dietary salt is an essential nutrient for the pregnant woman. It is required for optimum human reproductive efficiency. To restrict salt is to court disaster.

Dr. Robinson, while proving this important point, did so at agonizing cost to the families whose babies died due to maternal salt and protein restriction. Mothers in the low-salt group saw twenty-four more of their babies die—babies who might have been born healthy and strong if their mothers had happened to come into the clinic on another day.

Despite these findings many researchers today continue to demand that more studies like this be done on pregnant humans. Not satisfied with the wealth of supporting evidence from animal experiments conducted over the past fifty years, they propose studying the effects of drug therapy, protein restriction, calorie restriction, vitamin restriction, mineral restriction, etc.—all for the purpose of "seeing what will happen"! Their demands for "control" and "experimental" groups of pregnant mothers is clearly inhumane in light of the tragic consequences of just this one study, completed nearly twenty years ago. Persisting in subjecting more pregnant women and their unborn to hazardous deprivation experiments, or refusing to improve the diets of "control" mothers known to be suffering nutritional deficiencies in their daily diets, is criminal. Because of mounting criticism of such projects from a few lone voices in the scientific community and the public at large, many American researchers associated with prestigious universities and international health agencies have moved their projects out of this country. A baby who dies or is damaged in Guatemala provokes less outcry than one whose life is taken in Boston.

Ruth Pike, a nutritionist at Pennsylvania State University, influenced by Robinson's work, decided to see if she could duplicate her findings in a highly controlled laboratory situation—using pregnant rats instead of human mothers as experimental subjects. Specifically, she wanted to describe changes in organs brought on by low-salt diets in pregnancy. Her experiments are significant because she did not restrict protein in the diets of the rats. Salt intake was the only variable in her two groups.

She described two specific effects. First, rat mothers who were salt-restricted gave birth to offspring of low birth weight. Second, rat mothers on low-salt diets evidenced profound changes in the cells of the kidneys and adrenals. Pike found that when she reintroduced salt to the diet three days before delivery, the rats did not exhibit these changes. The damage to the organs was reversed when salt was added back to the diet.

She also observed that rats whose diets contained little salt and who were presented with containers of salt water and distilled water at the same time chose the salt water first. Only after drinking enough of the salt water to provide the necessary amount of salt for their normal body functions did the rats move to the distilled water. Pike's observations should have been brought to the attention of American obstetricians long ago by ACOG. Such an action would have convinced physicians to stop handing out low-salt diets to their pregnant patients as a matter of course.

Ranchers, farmers and veterinarians have arrived at the same conclusions as Robinson and Pike through their own experience and experiments. This 1968 reminder in the *Dairy Goat Journal* emphasizes their practical approach to the question of dietary salt:

> Salt is in the forefront of all feed additives. Both sodium and chloride, salt's two components, are needed in the nutrition and physiology of all animals, including man.
> Without salt, life as we know it could not exist. With too little salt in the diet, depending merely on the small amounts

of sodium and chloride inherently present in feeds, animals become unthrifty and in time go to pieces. Cows deliver weak calves, or even lose their calves. Cows actually die from salt starvation.

Researchers and people who work with animals would never presume to add a certain prescribed amount of salt to an animal's feed each day as a way of meeting that animal's needs. They follow the proven principle of allowing the animal's instinct for salt to operate. They set out salt blocks or buckets of crushed salt which the animals are free to lick as they feel the need. In this way, each animal's *individual needs* for salt are best met.

Humans have an identical salt-regulating mechanism which, when allowed to function, guarantees an adequate supply of salt to the body. Taste buds sensitive to salt are present on the tongue and inside the cheeks. When your body needs salt, your food tastes flat and unappetizing. This is a signal to add more salt to your food. In this simple way, nature alerts all of us to our metabolic needs for salt.

Should a person happen to take in more salt on a given day than she needs, a second salt-regulating mechanism is activated. Her kidneys respond automatically to the elevated salt concentration in the blood by allowing excess salt to leave the body in the urine. This built-in adjustment makes sure her body never becomes overloaded with salt.

Dr. Mary Jane Gray of the OB/GYN department of the University of Vermont Medical School has tested this salt-regulating mechanism in pregnant women. She tried to induce salt-overload in them and failed. Twenty-eight pregnant women were divided into two groups and followed for a month. Even with urging from the doctor to increase salt intake by means of salt tablets, capsules and syrups, the high-salt mothers retained no excess sodium in their bodies. Nor did any of them develop toxemia, although classic teaching has been that too much salt in the diet leads to toxemia.

There are a few medical conditions for which the standard treatment includes salt restriction. High blood pressure (hypertension), heart failure and kidney failure are examples. When women with such conditions become pregnant, or when pregnant women develop such conditions, special care must be exercised by the physician to see that the mother obtains enough salt to allow her blood volume to expand normally without triggering undesirable side effects. In the case of hypertension, recent research challenges the conventional wisdom. Dr. Lionel Schewitz of Michael Reese Hospital in Chicago reported in 1971 that even mothers with severe hypertension did better with liberal salt intake during pregnancy than when they were placed on rigid salt restriction and diuretics.

Otherwise healthy pregnant women may encounter some circumstances in which, though their kidneys are functioning normally, they may lose more salt from the body than is healthful. Many women report bouts of vomiting for a time during pregnancy, commonly during the first three months. Diarrhea from flu or other illnesses also results in excess loss of salt and water from the body. Or, if the mother lives in a hot climate, exercises strenuously, or works in a factory or laundry in high temperatures, she may sweat profusely. All these conditions boost the body's need for salt. If the mother does not take in more, salt-depletion will activate temporary salt-conserving mechanisms in the kidneys and adrenal glands. If salt deprivation continues, these organs can become exhausted and show signs of degenerative disease. The best way for each pregnant woman to be assured of meeting her individualized needs for salt is to follow the wisdom of the body and salt her food to taste throughout pregnancy. The body's simplest salt-regulating mechanism, the taste buds, are the most reliable guides to managing this aspect of human pregnancy nutrition.

Why, then, do doctors continue to place mothers on low-salt diets? Firmly fixed in their minds is the "magic number" they have erroneously accepted as the upper limit of safety for pregnancy weight gain—twenty-four pounds. Exceed twenty-four and risk toxemia, difficult labor and maybe a lifetime of obesity. When their thinking is dominated by these concerns, physicians are likely to accept any practice that seems to control weight—even that of restricting one of the most vital substances in the body—salt. It seems unlikely that the laws of physiology and biochemistry which govern human salt metabolism are suspended in the case of the pregnant woman. Yet doctors ignore these fundamental needs, and persist in viewing salt restriction as an easy, safe way to rid the mother of worrisome pounds.

The pregnant woman's problem is that her doctor has set *artificial standards* for weight gain and salt intake. In order to enforce these standards, he relies on her cooperation in a deliberate strategy of nutritional deprivation for the duration of her pregnancy. If she follows the diet, the protein-calorie deficiency it engenders will be further complicated by salt deficiency. After a time, her metabolism will be markedly altered due to physiologic stress caused by malnutrition. She will become ill. Her baby will suffer. The diet will have failed.

The low-salt, low-calorie diet doesn't work because it overlooks the body's physiologic salt-conserving mechanisms and brings about the very conditions it was designed to prevent:

1. High blood pressure: when salt is restricted below body requirements, the kidney reacts by releasing a hormone, renin, into the bloodstream. Renin influences other hormones which, in turn, cause the arterioles to constrict. The effect is to raise the blood pressure since the same

amount of blood is being pumped with the same force through a smaller opening. The obstetrician worries about high blood pressure (hypertension) since it often accompanies one of the most dangerous pregnancy diseases, toxemia. By putting the mother on a low-salt diet he is inducing hypertension where there was none before.

2. Low-protein intake: not only does the conventional low-salt, low-calorie diet directly limit the amount of protein available for the baby's growth and the mother's health by cutting back on her needed calories by one-third, but the low-salt provision sharply limits her range of food choices and makes the permitted foods less palatable. Her appetite wanes, so she will probably eat less than she could under the diet's rules. She will then be even more severely malnourished than a first look at the diet indicates. As her intake of protein falls, her liver becomes less able to manufacture circulating serum proteins, such as albumin, and albumin levels start to fall. As a result, water is lost from her bloodstream into the area surrounding the cells (interstitial space) and it appears that other substances in the blood, such as iron, are present in very high levels. Fluid lost from the bloodstream shows up as generalized swelling of tissues called edema. Edema caused by this fall in albumin levels is abnormal, a sign of disease (pathological). It is also associated with metabolic toxemia.

3. "Excess" weight gain: the edema will increase as long as the woman's body is malnourished. Her kidneys excrete less water in the urine as they scramble to keep salt and water concentrations in the body within normal limits; the reabsorbed water cannot be held in the bloodstream

since albumin levels are too low, so it leaks out into the tissues. Result: added swelling and added pounds.

A logical, effective alternative to this type of stopgap dietary meddling would be a program for pregnancy nutrition which respects physiology.

In order for an obstetrician to implement such a program in his practice, he would have to abandon traditional thinking and unscientific practices taught him by his professors in medical school. Instead, he would focus his efforts on preventive care—on getting each prospective mother to eat good foods to appetite and to salt her food to taste.

Doing so, though, would soon lead him to a confrontation with another aspect of his routine practice, the diagnosis and treatment of edema, or swelling. He would find, to his acute distress, that the vast majority of pregnant women who eat to appetite and salt to taste, whose diets provide the optimum amounts of protein, calories and salt, do swell during pregnancy—normally!

5

UNDERSTANDING SWELLING:
water retention is normal

Eighty to ninety percent of women swell up at some time in the course of their pregnancies. Most American obstetricians look on this normal swelling with alarm. The spectre of toxemia is never far from their minds, and toxemic women swell up.

Physicians have been trained to view swelling as a potential danger sign. When they see swelling of the face or hands, they recoil in horror. This is definitely a "condition" to be "treated." They attack the swelling with therapeutic frenzy. They de-salt. They drug. They dehydrate. Then they are confounded when their patients develop toxemia, anyway.

Dr. Leon Chesley, distinguished author of the toxemia chapter in *Williams Obstetrics,* the most widely used obstetrics textbook, now challenges this traditional approach to pregnancy swelling. After forty years of research in the field, he has concluded that normal swelling, or physiologic edema, is a sign of health in pregnant women, and not a pathological condition.

At a July 17, 1975, hearing of the Food and Drug Administration on the use of "water pills," or diuretics, in pregnancy, Dr. Chesley testified that 60 to 70 percent of normal pregnant women will have benign swelling of their faces and hands—in addition to that of their feet and ankles.[1]

This single statement is of enormous significance because up to two million pregnant women a year since 1958 have been placed on potent diuretics to "treat" the very edema Professor Chesley termed normal.

Citing study after study, going back as far as Dexter and Weiss's classic book on toxemia (1941), Dr. Chesley criticized the routine American obstetrical practice of "treating" pregnancy edema at all. Instead, he argued for an appreciation of its underlying physiologic causes.

Normal water retention comes about in pregnancy chiefly from an impressive rise in the level of female hormones, principally estrogens, manufactured by the placenta. These hormones are the same ones which cause many women to have water build-up and swelling in the few days preceding their menstrual periods, or when they are taking birth control pills. During pregnancy these hormones influence connective tissue throughout the body to retain extra fluid. Hence, the pregnant women commonly experiences swelling of her face and hands (generalized edema) in addition to that of her feet and lower legs (dependent edema).

The retained fluid is of benefit to mother and baby. Like a reservoir, it provides a water storage system in the mother's body. The stored fluid serves as a safeguard, a backup for the expanded blood volume we have learned is needed to nourish the placenta. At the time of birth, when some blood loss is unavoidable, the extra fluid protects the mother from going into shock. Remaining tissue fluid is mobilized in the early breast-feeding period to insure the mother an adequate milk flow.

---

[1] A complete transcript is available from: FDA, Bureau of Drugs, 5600 Fishers Lane, Rockville, MD 20852.

In women pregnant with twins, the process of physiologic swelling is exaggerated. Their larger placentas manufacture more hormones, which cause more water to be retained in their bodies—normally! This additional water, plus the weight of the second baby, dramatically increases the weight gain of the mother carrying twins. Weight gains of fifty to sixty pounds are typical when mothers are encouraged to eat well. Unfortunately, in the United States, where rigid weight control, salt restriction and diuretic therapy have characterized standard prenatal care, diagnosis of a twin pregnancy automatically assigns a mother to the so-called "high-risk" category. It is easy to understand why twins have had so much trouble when their intrauterine growth has been consistently subverted by these practices. It has even come to be accepted by doctors and mothers alike that "twins come early"—that they are born three or four weeks ahead of time, and that each must weigh less at birth than a single infant would. People have the idea that the mother's uterus had stretched as much as it could—"there was no more room"—so the babies had to be born.

When mothers of twins are counseled to eat correctly for three throughout gestation they meet their increased nutritional demands. When they refuse diuretics and low-salt diets for their extra physiologic edema they usually give birth, at term, to infants of normal birth weight. Twins are not of necessity "high-risk." They only become so when management incompatible with physiology is imposed by the physician.

Dr. Chesley, in his FDA testimony, consistently associated the presence of physiologic edema with better infant outcome. On two critical measures, birth weight and infant mortality, mothers with normal swelling did far better than those without it.

Drawing attention to a major conclusion of the 1968 *NIH Collaborative Study of Cerebral Palsy*, Dr. Chesley noted that babies born to mothers with normal swelling were of higher birth weight than those born to mothers with no swelling.

The Collaborative Study also found that a baby's birth weight is the most reliable indicator of future neurologic development. Low-birth-weight babies have a much higher likelihood of starting life with significant brain damage or growing up to face learning difficulties in school.

Dr. Chesley also reported a review of the medical records of 17,000 American mothers pregnant for the first time. In this study edema was associated not only with higher birth weight, but also with lower infant mortality. In 10,126 mothers who at no time had edema of the hands or face, the infant death rate was 26 per thousand. In the 6,963 mothers who did have edema of hands and/or face, the infant death rate was 18 per thousand. There was 44 percent higher infant mortality in the no-edema group!

After presenting this evidence and a very erudite discussion of the other harmful effects of "water pills" (which called into question the validity of the research which had originally persuaded the FDA to allow them to be used in pregnant women), Dr. Chesley went on record in opposition to the use of diuretics in human pregnancy. He stipulated only one exception to the blanket contra-indication. Diuretics may appropriately be used when the mother suffers heart failure, kidney malfunction, or other medical disease which results in abnormal water retention in both the tissues *and the circulation*.

This exception does not apply to toxemia, Dr. Chesley asserted. He adamantly stated that diuretics do not prevent or ameliorate toxemia. This bold conclusion discredited the slick, four-color spreads promoting diuretics which have appeared in every American OB/GYN journal since 1958. To the contrary, Dr. Chesley blamed diuretics for aggravating a significant abnormality present in mothers with toxemia, low blood volume (hypovolemia). The diuretics act to drive salt and water from the circulation, thus shrinking the blood volume even more. When used in conjunction with a low-salt diet from early pregnancy on, as the drug companies urged in their promotions, the diuretics may actually bring on the toxemia the doctor seeks to prevent.

What has been the outcome of this hearing? Up to now, most practicing obstetricians do not even know it was held. No testimony from the several physicians who appeared at the hearing has been publicized. The FDA has not called a public press conference to warn the public directly about the hazards of these drugs, even though millions of women and unborn babies continue to be exposed to them. Nor have the customary warnings been sent to physicians as was done recently after the disclosures that certain hormones often used to prevent spontaneous abortions cause vaginal cancer in female children born to mothers who took them in early pregnancy. Rather, the FDA has merely issued regulations requiring a change of labeling on the drugs, removing the indication that they are effective in toxemia. Most obstetricians practicing today have been trained to use these drugs as part of routine pregnancy management. Without special warnings, this labeling change in the fine print of the doctors' portion of the package insert will probably go unnoticed by the busy physician. Alarmingly, the American College of Obstetricians and Gynecologists, whose representative at the hearing argued that the drugs should continue to be prescribed if the mother is "too uncomfortable" at the end of pregnancy due to edema, still clings to this position. As a result, many thousands of women each year will continue to take these drugs because their doctors will continue to write the prescriptions.

Without the correct information from their physicians about

normal swelling, many women are dismayed by the way they look when they begin to swell a bit. Many physicians play on the mother's glum assessment of her looks as a way of forcing compliance with their low-salt diets and diuretics. If the mother refuses to cooperate, other forms of pressure may ensue. She is often told that her swelling is related to unnecessary accumulation of fat during pregnancy which will lead to permanent obesity. Or that her husband might lose interest in her if she becomes obese. The mother, not realizing that her swelling is probably normal and will vanish after the baby is born, accepts her doctor's appraisal.

One suburban mother angrily recalls how her obstetrician was so disgusted with her twenty-eight-pound weight gain and open disregard for his diet during her second pregnancy that he refused, point blank, to attend her delivery. He "taught her a lesson" by leaving her in the hands of an inexperienced resident she had never met before!

Her healthy baby boy weighed seven pounds—a marked difference from her first child, who weighed three and a quarter pounds and was born prematurely after an induced labor due to toxemia. This mother had followed the doctor's diet the first time, and the child has had an endless series of health problems since birth, a victim of intrauterine malnutrition.

Popular women's magazines stacked in the doctor's waiting room are of no help, either. Their pages are full of advertisements for mild diuretics to relieve swelling before a woman's period, or for "quick weight loss" when her favorite dress is a little too tight. Diet soda and junk food layouts promise satisfaction without nutrition. A barrage of underweight models promote emaciation as the American standard of beauty. Each issue rhapsodizes over the latest Hollywood diet guaranteed to keep readers vibrant and sexy while subsisting on only grapefruit, only rice, or only fluids. Little wonder the pregnant woman is on the defensive about her size and shape for nine straight months! No wonder she worries about swelling.

When swelling becomes uncomfortable, as it might toward the end of the pregnancy, the mother should take the following steps:

1. Switch to open, flat shoes like summer sandals. Feet are then free to swell as the day goes on, not pinched tight in closed shoes.

2. Try to minimize chair-sitting, especially on hard surfaces. Return of blood from the lower legs is impeded as the chair edge presses into upper leg. Sitting tailor-style (cross-legged) or using an ottoman for a footrest brings lower legs even with hips, assisting the flow of blood.

3. Lie with feet elevated on pillows, permitting return of blood pooled in feet and lower legs. Repeat three or four times a day, five to ten minutes each time.

4. Remove too-tight rings from swollen fingers.

5. Keep salting food to taste. Swelling can result from too little salt in the diet.

If the doctor suggests diuretics at any time in pregnancy, the mother must ask questions.

First, of herself: Am I eating a good, balanced diet for pregnancy? Am I getting enough protein, calories and salt? Swelling can result from deficiencies of any of these nutrients.

Next, of the doctor: Do I have any medical disease which causes an abnormal increase in blood volume, such as heart failure or nephritis? Diseases in which excess fluid is retained *in the circulation* may be aided by judicious diuretic therapy. An internist should be consulted and careful evaluation of the mother's condition made if any of these medical diseases are suspected. The good obstetrician recognizes his limitations and will seek consultation from other specialists when indicated.

Women must know that these diseases are exceedingly rare during the childbearing years. So rare, in fact, that if a doctor prescribes a diuretic for her, she must ask why she needs it. If he assures her she has no abnormal increase in her blood volume due to underlying medical disease, she should refuse to take the pills. Diuretics can do nothing but harm except in these rare situations.

Dr. Douglas R. Shanklin, professor in both the departments of OB/GYN and Pathology at the University of Chicago Medical School and past editor of the *Journal of Reproductive Medicine,* declared in 1973:

> Modern renal physiology makes it clear that the use of diuretics in pregnancy has little or no basis. There is a strong body of belief that they are causative of complications. The use of diuretics in pregnancy should be banned; they should be abandoned in modern prenatal care.

6

METABOLIC TOXEMIA
OF LATE PREGNANCY:
a disease of malnutrition

"**D**octor, it's Mrs. Gilbert on line two. She insisted on speaking to you."

Dr. Finley excused himself from his patient and took Eve's call in his private office.

"Hello, Doctor, I don't know exactly what's wrong. Everything's been going so well with the diet up until now, but this morning I can't get my feet in my shoes and my rings have gotten so tight I can't get them off. Also, the past two days I've been very tired. Last night Dick had to fix dinner when he came home. I didn't even feel like eating—and this morning I felt nauseated, too. I just got out of bed to call you. I know my regular appointment isn't until next week, but I was wondering if you could see me sometime today . . . if you could squeeze me in?"

Finley pulled Eve's chart from the file next to his desk.

"I see you were in last week, Eve. How long have you been following the diet?"

"Three weeks."

"And you've really been keeping with it? No deviations or substitutions?"

"Oh, no, Doctor. I've been cooking my food separately and letting Dick do the shopping so I won't snack on potato chips while I'm at the market. I admit I still want to use salt on things, but I know how important it is to control my weight right now . . . and that's the other thing that bothers me."

"Yes?"

"I think I've gained seven pounds this week. I don't know how, though. What do you think is wrong? I'm scared, Dr. Finley."

"Now don't worry, Eve. We can take care of this just fine. I want you to come in at one o'clock this afternoon. I'll check your blood pressure and take a look at this swelling and weigh you on our scales. It may just be a difference between your scales and ours that's upsetting you . . ." His voice trailed off.

"But I feel so weak—and look so puffy. Dick says I look like I got back all my baby fat. Should I have him come with me this afternoon?"

"Well, I don't think that will be necessary, Eve. If the swelling looks as bad to me as you say, we can give you some water pills to get rid of it in no time. I have some samples right here and you can get the prescription filled on your way home, okay?"

"But what if it's something else, what if it's toxemia?"

Toxemia of pregnancy, "the ancient enigma of obstetrics," has presented a grave danger to pregnant women throughout history. Hippocrates, the ancient Egyptians and the Chinese were perplexed by it.

Later medical writers observed that pregnant women with toxemia swell dramatically in the last half of pregnancy, gain large amounts of weight suddenly, develop high blood pressure and experience blinding headaches. Protein appears in their urine. In the most severe cases, women fall over in convulsions, lapse into coma and die, often with their babies undelivered.

Nobody knew why, though many theories were advanced to

explain the origin of this killer disease. Atmospheric conditions, emotional instability, a too-tight uterus in first pregnancies or twins, poisons from the breasts and fatty accumulations pressing on pelvic arteries have all been blamed at one time or another. Yet none of these theories has been able to account for all known cases.

Various treatments have been devised to combat the classic signs and symptoms known as the "toxemia syndrome." Low-salt diets and diuretics aimed at reducing swelling, low-protein diets aimed at stopping protein spills in the urine, low-calorie diets and amphetamines aimed at limiting weight gain, drugs aimed at lowering high blood pressure, drugs aimed at preventing convulsions and, as a last resort, delivery as soon as possible by inducing labor with synthetic hormones or by Caesarean section have all been tried. None of these therapies has successfully eliminated the disease because none has been directed at its underlying cause.

Today, as a result of evidence gathered by researchers over the past forty years, we know conclusively why pregnant women get toxemia. Even better, we know there is an inexpensive way to prevent toxemia in every pregnant woman.

A demonstration toxemia prevention project was instituted in the prenatal clinics of Contra Costa County, California, in 1963. During the twelve and one-half years of the project, Tom supervised the prenatal management of over seven thousand mothers from the lowest income group in the San Francisco Bay area. Over half the mothers belonged to ethnic minorities—Black, Mexican, American Indian and Oriental. Two-thirds of those having their first babies were teen-agers. All of these factors—poverty, race, age and number of pregnancies—contribute to what medical statisticians call a "high-risk" obstetrical population. These mothers, by all odds, should have had a great deal of trouble giving birth to healthy babies. They are considered to be especially likely candidates for developing toxemia and having low-birth-weight babies.

For example, during this period the university teaching hospital in Dallas reported that the toxemia rate in Black teen-age mothers delivering there was 35 percent. At Jacobi Hospital in New York City the estimated figure was 20 percent of all mothers having first babies. A rising maternal death rate from convulsive toxemia was reported by Dr. Lester Hibbard at Los Angeles County Hospital in 1973.

Unlike these other situations, the incidence of toxemia among mothers in the Contra Costa County project was 0.5 percent, with no cases reaching the convulsive stage.

What made the difference?

We credit four major changes made in daily clinical practices:

1. Redefining toxemia in a way that explained all cases;
2. Properly interpreting the classic signs of toxemia and refraining from merely treating them symptomatically;
3. Requiring that every mother attend nutrition counseling sessions with Tom;
4. Developing skills of communicating with mothers so they would understand and be motivated to follow the clinic nutrition program.

These departures from traditional methods were not easy to make. They evolved over a thirteen-year period of study and work in our southern states, the "eclampsia belt," so-called because of its persistently high rate of convulsive toxemia. Over these years it became necessary to rethink and reject much of what had become standard medical school teaching about the origin of the disease and its treatment.

Conclusions resulting from this laboratory and clinical research were published in 1966 in a handbook for the practicing physician, *Metabolic Toxemia of Late Pregnancy: a Disease of Malnutrition.*[1] In it a separate disease entity of known origin, metabolic toxemia of late pregnancy (MTLP), was differentiated for the first time from the "toxemia syndrome"—the well-known signs and symptoms associated with the disease. The clue to this discovery was the realization that the signs and symptoms which accompany MTLP can also be caused by other conditions. Sorting out which conditions are responsible for which aspects of the "toxemia syndrome" in any individual case is a process called differential diagnosis. Undertaking differential diagnosis whenever a mother displayed the "toxemia syndrome" was not taught in medical school or OB/GYN residency programs in the past—nor is it now.

The prevailing teaching has been that the "toxemia syndrome" (also known as "pre-eclampsia/eclampsia") is a disease of hypertension and kidney malfunction precipitated by an unknown underlying mechanism. This theory provided the physician no tools for use in the face of impending "toxemia," and, since the cause was officially unknown, every pregnant woman has been managed as though she were likely to develop the illness. If the signs and symptoms arose, all the physician could do was institute one of the myriad therapies and hope for the best. Lacking knowledge of the underlying cause of the disease, there could be no efforts at true prevention.

The book advanced a simpler thesis which gave the obstetrician a clear course of action to take in preventing the disease. The major conclusion was that fundamental disturbances in metabolism, chiefly in liver cells, afflicted mothers with MTLP. These

[1] Tom Brewer, M.D., Charles C. Thomas Publishers, Springfield, IL.

disturbances were caused by malnutrition and resulted in a malfunctioning liver. Thus, the "toxemia syndrome" of swelling, hypertension, protein in the urine and sudden weight gain must be viewed as the end result of metabolic derangement.

Characteristic liver lesions have been observed by pathologists for many years in mothers who have died of convulsive MTLP (eclampsia). In 1973 Sheehan and Lynch, two of England's leading pathologists, published a monumental review (1,719 references) of the world's literature on certain fatal diseases related to human pregnancy, including their own thorough autopsy reports on 677 obstetric patients. In 377 of these cases the mother had been suffering from "toxaemia of pregnancy." Sheehan and Lynch described specific changes in the livers of these mothers *which occur in no other recognized human disease.* Sometimes these lesions are so severe that they cause rupture of the liver and intra-abdominal hemorrhage. Tom pointed out in his book that similar liver lesions have been produced experimentally in animals deprived of proteins and other essential nutrients during gestation. In areas of the world where malnutrition is widespread, liver ruptures resulting from MTLP are often reported.

While malnutrition has been an undeniable fact of life for women living in poverty throughout history, the swing in 1958 in American obstetrical practice to rigid weight control, salt restriction and diuretic therapy as methods of routine pregnancy management made malnutrition an ever-present threat to women *in every economic group* who followed such dietary prescriptions.

It became clear that preventing malnutrition is the key to preventing MTLP. The successful Contra Costa County project was based on this single idea.

As Tom explains, "My interest in MTLP began in 1950 when I was a medical student at Tulane University Medical School, rotating through the OB/GYN department. One of the instructors, Dr. James Henry Ferguson, had spent the years 1946 to 1948 studying maternal deaths and the nutrition of pregnant women in rural Mississippi. He included material from his field work in his lectures. Our obstetrics textbook mentioned a new 'nutritional' theory of the origin of toxemia based on work done by Maurice Strauss and Bertha Burke at Harvard and Ferguson's research seemed to confirm it."

Toxemia was the number one cause of maternal death at that time throughout the South. In Mississippi seventy-six deaths from toxemia were reported in the first year of Ferguson's study. Rather than pore over medical records and state health department statistics, Ferguson chose a more direct way of finding out the conditions under which these unfortunate women had lived and died. He visited physicians and midwives who had had contact with a maternal death. He consulted public health nurses for information on the victim's background, home and diet. He visited some of their homes and personally interviewed over four hundred pregnant women coming to prenatal clinics in public hospitals. The picture that emerged was not a pretty one, nor one most well-fed and prosperous American physicians could accept as reality.

As Ferguson reported in the *Journal of the American Medical Association* in 1951:

> The case reports in this study are heavily weighted with women who are poverty stricken. Seventy-nine percent of these women can be classified as being in the lowest socioeconomic group.

He also published reports on the nutrition of the clinic patients he interviewed. Examples of some of the worst menus he encountered were:

I

Breakfast: 3 tablespoons grits
1 tablespoon butter
2 pieces of toast
1 cup coffee

Lunch: 1 candy bar
1 apple
1 soft drink

No dinner

II

No breakfast

Lunch: 1 root beer
2 plates field peas
4 biscuits (large)

Dinner: ½ plate water gravy
1½ plates fried okra
2 biscuits (large)

He found 94 percent of these mothers to be obviously malnourished: their diets were deficient in high quality proteins, iron, vitamin C, the B vitamins, calcium and many other nutrients recognized as essential. Eighty-nine percent did not receive a quart of milk a day and 57 percent had no eggs. More expensive sources of protein, such as lean meats, were way beyond their means.

The same miserable circumstances existed on the "toxemia ward" at Charity Hospital, Tulane's teaching institution serving the "medically indigent" from New Orleans and referrals from across Louisiana and Mississippi. The importance of taking in-depth histories detailing the life and dietary habits of the patient before entering the hospital was stressed in the internal medicine department.

Tom found, however, that on the OB/GYN service such histories were rarely taken. With over one thousand deliveries a month, 19 percent of which were complicated by the "toxemia syndrome," much of the patient care was on a strictly emergency basis. Only in the occasional case involving an internal medicine consultation was a detailed medical history attached to the patient's chart. The failure to take dietary histories on mothers admitted for "toxemia" denied the obstetricians an important clue to the underlying cause of the disease. It is impossible to get the right answers without asking the right questions. This missed opportunity left the doctors functioning in a vacuum. The only reality was the possibility that at any moment any one of the critically ill mothers on the ward might convulse.

One of the students' jobs was to go from bed to bed checking and recording the toxemic patients' blood pressures. As Ferguson had done in Mississippi, Tom asked the mothers what they had been eating before their admission to the hospital. They often volunteered that they had been vomiting for weeks off and on, then severely for a few days just prior to being hospitalized. Most were in the last trimester of pregnancy. The conversation:

"Did you have milk?"

"No, sir."

"Did you have eggs?"

"No, sir."

"Did you have meat?"

"Yes, sir."

"What kind of meat?"

"Fatback."

"Sow belly."

"Salt pork."

"Any lean meat?"

"No, sir."

Cornbread, grits, water gravy and field peas often constituted the rest of the diet.

In the crisis treatment center which was the "toxemia ward" in particular and the obstetrics service in general, the idea that malnutrition might be the cause of the problem was the farthest thing from the chief resident's mind.

It was his responsibility to supervise the anxious watch for convulsions, a sign that the disease had reached life-threatening proportions. The most important thing, when faced with rows of beds filled with patients who might convulse at any moment, was to ward off those convulsions! Repeated injections of mercury diuretics, magnesium sulfate and morphine had to be given in hopes of reducing gross swelling and achieving adequate sedation.

Trying to introduce the subject of meat, milk and eggs in this highly charged atmosphere must have seemed preposterous. At this late stage in the course of full-blown MTLP, any consideration of underlying cause appeared to be a speculative, academic matter. Even if anyone knew the cause, by the time the seriously toxemic mother reached the ward there was nothing to be done about the disease but treat it. Prevention was simply not part of the thinking of the time.

Tom recalls: "That goal became very important in my own professional life, but to prevent the disease, I had to learn more about it. In particular I wanted to find out what biochemical events, for instance, preceded the liver damage so many investigators reported associated with convulsive toxemia."

Thousands of hours spent pouring over scientific reports in *Chemical Abstracts* yielded little. Virtually every biochemical test known had been done on normal pregnant women and those with the "toxemia syndrome," but confusion was rampant. Conflicting results on the same tests done on the same populations in different medical centers were the rule. Clearly the researchers were not all calling the same set of phenomena by the same name, or there were variables in their samples of which they were unaware.

During his internship at the city-county hospital in Houston, Tom noticed that the private attending physicians seemed not to worry about "toxemia." They often commented, "We have to come over here to Jeff Davis to see pre-eclampsia, eclampsia and abruptions of the placenta. We don't see these in private practice."

Tom notes: "Their remarks strengthened my growing belief that MTLP historically afflicted the poor because the poor were more likely to be malnourished. From 1955 to '58 in my private general practice in Fulton, Missouri, I saw no cases of MTLP in one hundred pregnancies. The absolute difference between the malnourished women of the 'toxemia wards' and this better-fed group of mothers confirmed what the Houston obstetricians had told me. MTLP was, at that time, a rare complication in middle-class women."

The subject came up occasionally during informal talks with other doctors in Fulton. They usually credited the absence of toxemia among their patients to the higher economic status and generally better health of the women in Fulton as compared to the women they had cared for in their training days. "Poverty" was the reason for all the troubles they had seen back in the inner city teaching hospitals. But the idea that poverty usually meant malnutrition and that malnutrition predisposed to disease never entered the conversation. The casual expectation of the doctors was that mothers who made up the bulk of private practice would go through pregnancy just fine and have a normal baby. The sharp contrast between this attitude and that which prevailed in the university centers helps explain a development in routine pregnancy management which in retrospect seems almost inconceivable.

A look at the medical journals of the 1950's and 1960's leaves little doubt as to which attitude gradually came to dominate the American OB/GYN consciousness and inadvertently lay the groundwork for middle-class pregnancy malnutrition on an unprecedented scale. The emphasis on pregnancy complications, crisis-management and drug therapies is so overwhelming that if one had no other source of information about pregnancy in mid-century America, one would be driven to conclude that it was a high-risk condition of the same order as impending heart attack. The journals reflect this point of view because they are written primarily by and for researchers in teaching institutions whose "material" for study is almost exclusively comprised of malnourished, poverty-stricken women who do indeed have many pregnancy problems.

Abetting the preoccupation with pregnancy pathology were drug company advertisements, each of which tried to outdo the others in convincing the physician of the efficacy of their products. Since claims made in these advertisements are based on research done in the university medical schools with grant money provided by the drug companies, it should not be surprising that journal articles and drug company promotions address the same concerns and reinforce each other's conclusions. Drug companies in this country, of course, are in business to make a profit. Advertising in medical journals is an important part of overall marketing strategy.

For thirty years competition in the pregnancy "market" has been focused on developing new ways of dealing with that old problem, weight control. Excess weight gain has been implicated for decades in the onset of toxemia, so, to the traditionally trained obstetrician, any assistance he can get in preventing un-

due weight gain he tends to view as an aid to preventing toxemia. The drug company market analysts know of the university
physicians' continual concern about toxemia, and their promotional campaigns ever since the late 1940's have featured advertisements in which the spectre of toxemia looms as an un-
spoken menace. By never allowing the obstetrician to forget the
"toxemia ward" of his training, a "market" is created for weight
control drugs which can only be obtained by prescription. Prescriptions mean profits.

The first category of drugs to be approved for use in pregnancy
weight control were appetite depressants (amphetamines or
"speed"). At first promoted primarily for mothers who were overweight at the beginning of pregnancy, they were quickly taken
up for use in enforcing rigid patterns of weight gain in normal
mothers as well. Competition for dominance in the lucrative pregnancy weight control "market" was keen. The July 15, 1962 issue
of the *American Journal of Obstetrics and Gynecology* probably
represents the pinnacle of corporate contention: four major drug
companies, each with full-page layouts.

In them we learn that Ambar Extentabs, a combination of amphetamine (an "upper") and phenobarbitol (a "downer")—later
in the ad described as a "balanced formula"—are "small . . .
easy to take . . . suppress appetite for up to 12 hours . . . improve
mood *without* 'jitters' . . . and help establish conservative eating
habits." With Tenuate, the doctor can "control weight gain from
test to term" by "suppressing appetite with no effect on heart
rate, blood pressure, pulse, respiration and no alteration of basal
metabolism rate (BMR)." The doctor might also consider Dexamyl
Spansule, a brand of sustained release capsules containing Dexe-
drine and amobarbital ("Warning, may be habit forming") especially effective "during pregnancy . . . to keep her weight right
and her outlook bright." For those who had a few pounds to lose

during pregnancy, the doctor could count on Desoxyn Gradu-
met, "the all-day appetite control from a single oral dose" which
caused side effects such as insomnia, nervousness and palpitation
in only 15 to 20 percent of patients!

These advertisements never pointed out that a mother could
be obese because her diet was high in carbohydrates, sugars and
fats and low in protein, vitamins and minerals. Nor was there ever
an intimation that a more appropriate form of physician intervention would be to switch the mother to a higher quality diet, instead
of counseling her to do anything she could to hold her weight down.
Because doctors had been trained to think of the baby as a parasite and "toxemia" as a consequence of excess weight gain, the
concept that dieting during pregnancy might be harmful to baby
and mother completely escaped them. During no phase of their
training had anyone made the link between malnutrition and
poor pregnancy outcome, so it was easy for them to be seduced
into prescribing amphetamines, unaware that reducing any mother's food intake below pregnancy requirements could harm the
baby. This major clinical error could only have come about as
the result of medical training which failed to take into account
the malnutrition of the poorest mothers in the country. If doctors
had fully recognized the role of malnutrition in human reproductive casualty, they could never have been induced to cooperate in
the next phase of maternal starvation for profit—the campaign for
sodium diuretics.

Capitalizing on their by-then well-established "market" for
pregnancy weight control, the major drug companies added a new
promotional twist in January 1958. With full approval of the Food
and Drug Administration, the American Medical Association
(AMA) and the American College of Obstetricians and Gynecologists (ACOG), a new category of drugs was introduced for
use in pregnancy—thiazide diuretics. The journal ads for the

thiazides displayed concern over one specific component of the "excess" weight gain targeted by the amphetamine ads, pregnancy swelling (edema). Since gross swelling is associated with severe toxemia, and responsible for the sudden increase in weight in toxemic mothers, the ads encouraged the physician to take charge of the situation as he had been trained to do on the "toxemia" ward. By prescribing a diuretic, the ads proclaimed, the doctor could "prevent pre-eclampsia or toxemia" and provide relief from the "discomfort of late pregnancy edema" without having to hospitalize the mother. Until this time, the most effective diuretic, mercury, had to be given by injection. Its use was of necessity limited to the critically ill who populated the "toxemia" wards.

With the advent of the thiazides, all that changed. Far more potent than any of their precursors, the thiazides acted directly on the kidney, effecting wholesale excretion of salt, water and potassium from the body. They were effective when taken by mouth, so even the mother on the most rigorous diuretic therapy could now maintain her customary activities.

Just as the amphetamine ads never acknowledged the different status of mothers who gained weight on sound diets from those who gained on poor diets, the ads for thiazides never distinguished between the multitude of conditions that could cause fluid retention in the pregnant woman. On the contrary, the ads give the impression that all edema is worth "treating"—and the sooner in pregnancy the better, so no serious problem could develop. Because doctors themselves had not been trained to differentiate between physiologic edema (which accompanies nearly every pregnancy to some degree) and pathological edema resulting from an underlying disease, all edema came to be viewed as suspect. Because edema is so common, the "market" for the new diuretics was much broader than that for amphetamines alone had been. Because edema can be associated with MTLP, doctors were interested in a drug which promised to help them eliminate this threat to their patients. Because few physicians reflected on the deleterious effects of interfering with the body's normal mechanisms governing salt metabolism, there was not a murmur of protest as drug companies took the position that all water retention is potentially harmful.

Sales of the thiazides zoomed as ten giants of the pharmaceutical industry engaged in a long-running battle for their share of the profit-laden "market." Huge advertising budgets were allotted to the diuretic campaign. Conferences, seminars and medical meetings, traditionally sponsored by drug manufacturers, were highlighted by attractive booths featuring the new diuretics and, as usual, the industry reached the physician in his office with its direct mail promotion and 35,000 company representatives, the "detail men."

In 1973, after certain studies showed that thiazides damaged mothers and babies, one major company voluntarily withdrew its promotions for its diuretic compound. The medical director of this firm disclosed that by the time the average drug hits the market, the company has spent five million dollars to develop it and that only after five years of intensive promotion will the product begin to make money. This often puts the company in the position of having to push the product even in the face of evidence that the drug might be harmful to the user. These economic imperatives account for the reluctance of the drug companies to remove the thiazides from the pregnancy "market." Not until the FDA acted in June of 1976 to require a labeling change on these drugs did the other nine firms in the diuretic business abandon their pregnancy promotions, despite the fact that reported side effects from the thiazides, as listed on the package for the doctor's information, ran the gamut of insults to mother and baby. Loss of appetite, stomach irritation, diarrhea, constipation, cramping, jaundice, pancreatitis, hyperglycemia, hypertension, dizziness, headache, thrombocytopenia, sugar in the urine, depression of bone marrow function and allergic reactions were noted.

In addition to these side effects of the drugs themselves, several of which—like loss of appetite—have direct bearing on the mother's nutritional status, the detail man carried with him an adjunct to diuretic therapy which made it even more hazardous: the low-salt, low-calorie diet sheet. The low-salt provision supposedly reduced the likelihood that a mother would retain excess sodium in her tissues, thereby heading off edema from the very start of pregnancy. The low-calorie provision kept alive the notion that weight control was necessary in the fight against "toxemia."

The diet sheets, several of which were authored by professors in prestigious departments of OB/GYN, were a great blow to the concept of sound nutrition in pregnancy. Because they, like the new diuretics, were intended to be used by every pregnant woman as a preventive measure against the onset of "toxemia," even the healthiest mother in the country would be exposed to the hazards of malnutrition if she followed the regimen. In the original research on the thiazides, mothers had been permitted to use as much salt as they wished while they were on experimental diuretic therapies. So, even though the thiazides depleted the body's supply of sodium, mothers could keep up with their requirements by taking in more. When the diuretics were used rigorously in conjunction with the low-salt diets, however, metabolic consequences were likely to be catastrophic. Not only would the mother have a much higher risk of developing MTLP, but her baby's rate of intrauterine growth would be slowed due to a reduced supply of blood to the placenta.

Estimates of how widespread the use of diuretics and low-salt diets became are mind-boggling. A survey conducted in 1963 in Tulsa, for instance, showed 93 percent of doctors responsible for prenatal care reporting that they used thiazide diuretics exactly as they had been promoted: in the treatment of edema, for weight control, and to treat and prevent "toxemia." Diuretic therapy became an accepted part of routine prenatal care in the United States and has been going strong ever since 1958. There is evidence that up to two million pregnant women a year have taken diuretics and even more mothers have been managed with salt restriction and weight control as essential, unquestioned practices.

Tom became deeply disturbed by the promotions for the thiazides when they first appeared in 1958. "I was convinced from my own experience and study," he relates, "that adoption of this approach to pregnancy management would *produce* MTLP, not prevent it. The malnutrition and dehydration resulting from the diet and drugs would make any woman subject to the same diseases and complications of pregnancy suffered by women in poverty for generations. In the case of the middle-class mother, though, this nutritional deprivation would be engendered by the advice of her physician. I decided to undertake further research to try to find a way to prevent MTLP. I was especially interested in the relationship between malnutrition and liver dysfunction since many researchers had called attention to certain liver lesions unique to patients with MTLP."

In his last year at Miami's Jackson Memorial Hospital, Tom became chief OB/GYN resident with the authority to test one of the results of his research: a new method of managing the mother acutely ill with MTLP.

There are two central problems presented by these patients. Solving each provided a strategy for true prevention of the conditions which precipitate MTLP. These mothers have markedly contracted blood volumes (hypovolemia) and they have impaired liver function due to malnutrition. Neither of these problems was taken into consideration by the standard protocol for treating "toxemia." With the advent of the more potent thiazide diuretics, the patient with hypovolemia was at even greater risk than before.

One of the earliest signs of developing MTLP is a fall in the serum albumin levels in the mother's blood. Albumin is a protein which keeps water in the circulation. It is manufactured by the liver. More albumin is required during pregnancy to maintain the normally expanded maternal blood volume. When the mother's diet is inadequate, the liver cannot synthesize enough albumin to keep up with the extra demands of pregnancy and albumin levels in the blood fall, allowing water which should be in the circulation to leak out into the mother's tissues. More significantly, her blood volume falls and the ability of the placenta to function starts to decrease.

Result: she appears swollen and puffy from the abnormal accumulation of water. The extra water retention also causes a sudden increase in weight.

During pregnancy the liver is working overtime to meet the stress of increased metabolic functions of all kinds. If the mother is malnourished in the last half of pregnancy, impairment of albumin synthesis can occur in a matter of weeks!

If the mother's diet is not improved, the blood volume continues to fall. Her body compensates in at least three ways:

1. the kidneys start to reabsorb water in an effort to restore fluid to the circulation. But without sufficient albumin, the reabsorbed water also leaks into the tissues, thus aggravating the edema;

2. blood pressure rises in an attempt to maintain adequate blood flow to all organs;

3. if blood volume becomes critically low, the kidneys shut down completely causing urinary output to dwindle to zero.

At this point in the traditional management of the severely toxemic patient, the answer has been to administer ever more potent diuretics to the mother in hopes of boosting her urinary output and reducing abnormal swelling.

In these circumstances, the diuretics are lethal. They act in the body only to remove more water from the already perilously shrunken blood volume. They are unable to affect the abnormal swelling because they do not contain any substance capable of attracting tissue fluid back into the circulation. Instead, they rob the patient of the very fluid she needs in her bloodstream to keep heart, lungs and brain functioning.

With repeated doses of the diuretics, the mother eventually lapses into hypovolemic shock: exactly the same condition as if she had been in an auto accident and were bleeding uncontrollably. In both cases the mother lacks enough blood to sustain normal body functions. Tom witnessed several maternal deaths in the hospital following such a course of diuretic therapy.

Later reports in the literature indicated that this phenomenon was widespread. Advocates of the new diuretics overlooked the problem of hypovolemia. They maintained it was the "toxemia" which killed the mother, not the drugs.

In one case in 1969, a Vallejo, California, mother with three previous normal pregnancies died of MTLP along with her unborn twins in a famous medical center. The family sued the physician for malpractice.

During the trial, the plaintiff's attorney entered in evidence drug company literature warning against using the most potent diuretics, Lasix and Edecrin, at any time in pregnancy. This woman had been given both drugs in the hospital to combat her swelling.

The doctor's defense: we all use these drugs, anyway. Five of his colleagues testified that the doctor had done all he could do and, despite his efforts, the mysterious "toxemia" had finally killed her. The treatment he gave was just what they all would have given. The jury found the doctor innocent.

Tom's new approach to the patient with MTLP involved giving the mother the substance her damaged liver could not synthesize—human serum albumin. If the theory were right, the woman's urinary output should markedly increase and her abnormal swelling should begin to disappear after administration of the albumin. This course of treatment would not heal her liver, but at least she would be spared hypovolemic shock and kidney shutdown.

It worked. Since then other researchers have confirmed his clinical trials. Dr. Peggy Howard of Chattanooga and Dr. Stella Cloren of Basel, Switzerland, working independently, have administered serum albumin to more than 175 mothers with MTLP. Their reports of excellent results lend weight to the original study.

The albumin experiment was gratifying because it linked liver impairment to the classic signs of MTLP. However, the primary goal was not to rescue women suffering from advanced MTLP, but to prove that *sound nutrition alone* could improve the conditions of mothers who were developing MTLP and prevent it completely in all other mothers if adopted as routine prenatal management.

Tom instituted an experimental dietary intervention program at Jackson Memorial which had several unconventional features:

First, mothers with MTLP were placed on a high-protein (120 grams per day) diet. Dr. Maurice B. Strauss, the Harvard internist, had shown thirty years before that high-protein diets improved the conditions of mothers with what he termed "nutritional toxemia."

Second, the mothers were placed on regular, rather than salt-restricted diets. A salt shaker appeared on the tray at each meal and the mother was instructed to salt her food to taste.

Third, the women were encouraged to stay out of bed as much as possible, even to do chores on the ward if they were willing, rather than being ordered to the customary bedrest.

Fourth, diuretics and drugs to lower blood pressures were not used.

Fifth, following the work of Poth on the most effective way to suppress bacterial flora in the bowel, patients received oral antibiotics to reduce the detoxication load on their damaged livers.

Sixth, Tom personally discussed the program with each mother to obtain her permission and cooperation, then made a conscientious effort to see that each followed her diet well.

Not every patient admitted to the hospital with the diagnosis of "toxemia" was accepted for the high-protein feeding program. Often after consultation and laboratory work, it would turn out that the mother did not have MTLP at all. Though she presented the same set of signs and symptoms—the "toxemia syndrome"—characteristic of MTLP, it was found she could have a problem totally unrelated to liver malfunction. For instance, physiologic edema, bladder and kidney infections, nephritis, chronic hypertension and obesity were often misdiagnosed as toxemia.

It became clear why other researchers had experienced such difficulty in understanding toxemia. Their definition had been imprecise, and even the simplest biochemical tests done on women with MTLP and women with nephritis, for example, turn up very divergent results.

Ten patients over two years met the program admission requirements. Nine improved, doing significantly better by all measures than women on traditional toxemia management.

The one mother who did not respond to the dietary program was carrying twins. She had made eight prenatal visits to the county clinic. At each visit she had complained about constant nausea and vomiting, but no steps were taken to help her correct it. As a consequence she had a very poor diet with low-protein intake. After nine days in the hospital, during which she was unable to eat an adequate diet, she spontaneously went into labor and gave birth to twins weighing three and a half and four pounds.

Tom observed: "This mother was so severely malnourished that her protein reserves had been depleted. After delivery and subsequent mobilization of her edema fluid, she weighed only 72 pounds (height 5 feet, 2 inches) and looked as if she had just come out of a concentration camp. Her liver had been so compromised by malnutrition that nothing short of delivery could initiate the healing process."

This result was encouraging because it showed that poor nutrition, not some mysterious substance manufactured by the placenta, was responsible for the onset of MTLP. Also significant was the fact that no mothers got worse after being placed on the program—a clear refutation of all those who claim that eating salt leads to toxemia, that eating to appetite results in excess weight gain which leads to toxemia, that diuretics must be given to prevent toxemia, that forced bed rest could improve the conditions of women with MTLP.

In 1963 Tom began the broad-based toxemia prevention project in the Contra Costa County prenatal clinics to which we have referred. He thought, "If MTLP can be eliminated among the group of mothers considered to be at greatest risk of developing the disease, then perhaps these nutritional methods would be tried and confirmed by others. These clinical tests of the approach, I hoped, would form the basis of a new set of standards for routine prenatal care which would be institutionalized all over the country."

The major innovation of the Contra Costa County project was the weekly nutrition seminar conducted with new clinic patients. The authority of the physician in charge was a crucial psychological factor in altering the behavior of the mothers in his care—especially in the culturally influenced area of food habits.

The informal discussion format encouraged mothers to ask questions and volunteer information about their past pregnancy experiences. In this way, mothers learned from one another as well as from the doctor what some of the hazards of malnutrition were. In addition to explaining the physiologic changes the mother could expect as pregnancy advanced, the importance of good nutrition in promoting these changes and facilitating an easier birth and postpartum period was stressed.

The unique feature, though, was reviewing how many common complications of pregnancy are concretely linked with poor nutrition. When mothers learned the consequences of malnutrition for themselves and their babies, they became serious about eating correctly. No supplemental foods were distributed at the clinic. Nutritional counseling *given by the physician* was the sole mode of dietary intervention.

At each follow-up visit with individual mothers, the initial educational talk was reinforced. During these conversations the mother could report on how well she was following the prescribed diet, discuss the problems she was having with it or ask any questions she might have. Every mother was reminded to continue to eat good foods to appetite and to salt her food to taste. No mention was made of weight gain, except in cases where underweight mothers were failing to gain.

In this situation, where the authority of the doctor was used to encourage sound nutritional habits and not to impose strict limits on weight gain, convulsive MTLP never once occurred in twelve and a half years, and mild MTLP was reduced to 0.5 percent.

As the Contra Costa County project progressed, Tom gradually became confident that the nutritional thesis of MTLP was correct. As is customary, he published journal articles about the project and began to lecture at medical meetings and hospitals around the country, urging obstetricians to try these methods and abandon those being promoted by pharmaceutical interests. He also started petitioning the FDA to hold a hearing on the use of diuretics and low-salt diets in pregnancy. This campaign was to take ten years to come to fruition.

As he traveled, he found that clinics everywhere were being run as they had been when he was a medical student in 1950 and an OB/GYN resident in 1960. Although some clinics had introduced dietary counseling provided by nutritionists, the authority of the doctor in charge almost always ran counter to their best efforts. One nutritionist from Mobile, Alabama, summed up her experience:

> It has been our major teaching point to emphasize foods high in protein—specifically, lean meats, milk and eggs. We have an interview with every patient on each maternity clinic visit to instruct her in normal nutrition.
>
> The nutritionists here have been confronted with conflicting ideologies concerning prenatal nutrition. The low-calorie, low-sodium, diuretic treatment is used by the majority of obstetricians. This has caused a head-on collision with the purpose of the nutritionists.

The Contra Costa project results confirmed those of Dr. Reginald Hamlin of Sydney, Australia, who, while chief of OB/GYN at the Crown Street Women's Hospital, also taught nutrition to clinic mothers from 1948 to 1951. For the preceding ten years there had been one case of convulsive MTLP in every 350 deliveries in his hospital. By the third year of his nutrition education efforts, there was not one case in 5,000 consecutive deliveries. As Hamlin expressed it, MTLP is caused by "a relative deficit of first class proteins and vitamins." He attributed his success to a program which "was aimed strategically at the occult basis of the disease instead of at its summit of classical late signs and symptoms." The result:

> The humicribs (incubators) were often empty now. By 1949 nurses and medical students were beginning to ask why they were no longer seeing enough eclamptics (patients with convulsive MTLP) . . . By 1950 it was felt that one could say to the skeptics: Eclampsia will no longer afflict the patients of this hospital if the present methods of prevention are followed meticulously.

Hamlin's remarkable work, like that of Strauss, Burke, Ferguson and others who linked MTLP with malnutrition, remains almost completely unknown in American obstetrics today.

The conclusion that MTLP is completely preventable by sound nutrition has been brushed aside in the rush to ever more farfetched therapies. In the 1960's it was diuretics which were going to prevent toxemia. Now, technological detection of fetal illness and warehousing of large numbers of "high-risk" mothers and babies in regional perinatal centers are the rage. Rarely in the academic centers does one hear or read of the protective effects of scientific nutrition during gestation. At a recent meeting of the International Federation of Obstetricians and Gynecologists, for instance, eighty papers were presented. Thirty of them dealt with fetal monitoring and its special applications in the "high-risk" case.

Examination of the current OB/GYN journals turns up the

same preoccupation with diagnosis and treatment of disease. Those investigators who write on toxemia spend years of their lives painstakingly measuring biochemical irregularities in mothers with the disease. Though they write copiously documented reports of their efforts, these researchers rarely say a word about prevention.

Since the bulk of practitioners continue to give traditional care when it comes to nutrition, a non-profit organization committed to the establishment of scientific standards of nutrition management in American obstetrics was founded in 1972, the Society for the Protection of the Unborn through Nutrition (SPUN). Only when official OB/GYN practice standards have been set for sound maternal nutrition will the idea become incorporated into medical school teaching. Until that time, *every* mother and *every* unborn baby will continue to be at risk from the known hazards of nutritional deprivation during pregnancy.

The issue of pregnancy nutrition management is also being addressed in the courts. In a precedent-setting decision in September 1977 an Indiana jury awarded a mentally retarded woman fifty thousand dollars in a malpractice suit that charged her mother's prescribed diet during pregnancy caused her retardation. A diet of polished white rice, fruit, and a daily dose of Epsom salts, plus shots of mercury diuretics, was prescribed for the mother during the last two months of her pregnancy for the treatment of toxemia. Expert witnesses for the family testified that the diet, because of its low protein content, caused the child's retardation.

Commenting editorially, the *Chicago Tribune* observed: "The jury's message is an urgent one to the medical profession . . . because it gives judicial recognition to the importance of proper nutrition during pregnancy." Jay Hodin, executive director of

SPUN, which assisted in the case by arranging for specialists' testimony, noted:

> The paucity of nutrition education in medical training by no means, the Indiana jury decided, relieves those obstetricians who impose inadequate diets upon expectant mothers from liability. The most significant outcome of the trial, and one whose implication is likely to reverberate throughout the medical community, is that malpractice may be construed to include obstetricians' casual attitudes toward nutrition in pregnancy. Many studies link inadequate prenatal diet to a wide range of newborn and childhood diseases and disorders.

SPUN maintains a National Toxemia/Intervention Hotline for women and professionals who wish to consult experts about possible cases of MTLP and its management: (914) 271-6474.

The Contra Costa County clinic project demonstrated that no mother who is able to eat, digest, absorb and metabolize a diet adequate for pregnancy will develop MTLP.

Whenever a mother in the project developed the "toxemia syndrome," one of two things was happening.

Either she was not following the diet.

Or she had something else.

7

"TOXEMIA" IN THE WELL-NOURISHED:
mistaken diagnosis

The majority of obstetricians dismiss the idea that malnutrition causes toxemia. Their reason: they have seen many patients who were well nourished and still displayed the signs and symptoms of the "toxemia syndrome." Therefore, toxemia, as they have traditionally thought about it, could not possibly result from malnutrition.

Their position sounds reasonable, but it is based on a common clinical error.

When confronted by a mother with the "toxemia syndrome," these physicians customarily skip the important process of differential diagnosis. Instead, they make a reflex diagnosis of toxemia whenever one or more of the classic signs is present: swelling of hands and face, excess weight gain, protein in the urine or elevated blood pressure. No further evaluation is deemed necessary.

The result: many thousands of pregnant women have been diagnosed as toxemic and treated for toxemia they did not have.

Serious problems result from this mistake. The mother with some other condition which appears similar to MTLP continues to suffer her original malady because it goes undiagnosed and untreated. Further, the mother may well develop MTLP as a result of the low-salt, low-calorie diet and drugs prescribed for her. She and the baby may develop further symptoms from prescribed diuretics, amphetamines and antihypertensives which cross the placenta.

Differential diagnosis is a routine practice in internal medicine. It means that the doctor carefully considers and selectively rules out different conditions which produce the same signs or symptoms in an individual case.

In order to make an accurate diagnosis of what is causing the "toxemia syndrome" in a given mother, the obstetrician must be persuaded to withhold judgment and treatment until all the possibilities have been examined, consultations with specialists in other medical disciplines have been undertaken and appropriate laboratory tests run whenever indicated.

Unfortunately, under current circumstances in which the obstetrician has not been trained to carry out differential diagnosis of the "toxemia syndrome," responsibility for insuring that an accurate diagnosis is made rests with the person least likely to know how to proceed—the mother herself! The mother who finds herself in this situation must realize that her prime responsibility is to her unborn baby. She must insist that the doctor follow through with a complete evaluation of her condition before deciding whether any form of therapy is warranted. If she is not satisfied with the doctor's performance, she must not feel disloyal or ungrateful about requesting a consultation with a specialist in the suspected area. If necessary, she should make such arrangements on her own and request of the office nurse that her *complete* records be sent to the consulting doctor. Her main concern is not to appease the doctor but to obtain clear, complete explanations of his medical decisions before she decides whether to take his advice.

In order to become her own advocate in this troublesome plight, the mother needs to know what conditions other than MTLP account for the most common signs and symptoms of the "toxemia syndrome." She must also be sure she does not have MTLP!

The first step is responsible evaluation of her diet. MTLP cannot be ruled out unless the mother is obtaining enough protein, calories, vitamins, minerals, salt and water to keep her liver and other organs functioning optimally throughout pregnancy. Unless someone has made a special point of giving her correct advice about pregnancy nutrition, she probably assumes her customary eating habits are satisfactory for pregnancy. The idea that pregnancy is a nutritional stress for *every* woman, regardless of her pre-pregnancy diet or economic status, is not widely held. Most mothers, if asked, reply that they eat well. They usually mean that they eat what they like! Consequently, nutritional nonchalance commonly affects mother and doctor alike.

To determine the true state of affairs, the mother has to consider what foods she has been eating recently and in what quantities. She should realize that flu or other gastrointestinal disturbances like nausea and vomiting interfere with her eating pattern. Her appetite may also suffer if she has been worried or depressed. Any of these conditions may result in malnutrition.

If her dietary evaluation shows she is well nourished, then MTLP can be ruled out and other explanations for the sign or symptom under consideration must be found.

A primer of mistaken diagnoses and how to avoid them is a distinct help to mother and physician.

Swelling of hands and face (generalized edema), as we have discussed, is probably the most commonly misdiagnosed sign. Sixty percent of normal pregnant women experience swelling of their hands and face as a manifestation of healthy adjustment in pregnancy—*if the mother is well nourished.* It does not require treatment of any kind at any time in pregnancy.

Protein in the urine commonly occurs in pregnant women who develop a *urinary tract infection,* either in the kidneys or the bladder. Pregnant women are more likely to develop such infections because of continual pressure on the tubes which drain the kidneys early and late in pregnancy. Simple urinalysis may not reveal the presence of infection, so a quantitative urine culture should be done to establish the correct diagnosis and appropriate medication to combat the infection.

Many types of *kidney disease,* such as glomerulonephritis (Bright's disease), chronic pyelonephritis, kidney cysts and tumors, also cause protein spills in the urine. Differentiation between the various kidney disorders is the specialty of the renal expert, who should be consulted by the obstetrician when these diseases are under consideration.

Elevated blood pressure (hypertension) may result from many different causes. "Psychic" hypertension, is engendered by *emotional stress* of any sort. Many women become anxious during physical examinations or during laboratory testing. Women whose blood pressure has been normal throughout pregnancy may develop hypertension at the time of admission to the hospital for labor and birth. These mothers do not have MTLP: the liver is functioning normally and the blood volume is expanded.

"Essential," chronic, or benign hypertension is most common in women over thirty years of age. However, many black teen-agers have already developed the condition and will continue to have it the rest of their lives. These mothers require exactly the same diet as mothers with normal blood pressures—including the use of salt to taste—since their blood volumes must expand, too, as pregnancy advances.

Salt deficiency can trigger hypertension as mentioned previously.

Obese women are often incorrectly diagnosed as hypertensive when a standard size blood pressure cuff is used to take a reading. When the cuff is too small, additional pressure on the mother's arm reads on the meter as elevated blood pressure. Using a larger cuff prevents this error.

Pheochromocytoma, an exceedingly rare tumor of the adrenal gland, also causes hypertension.

Kidney diseases also result in high blood pressure.

Other signs—pregnant women may develop medical diseases that afflict the rest of the population: epilepsy, brain tumor, stroke, heart failure, cirrhosis of the liver and poorly controlled diabetes mellitus may also be included in the differential diagnosis if the preceding conditions yield no answers.

Obviously, what was once considered a simple clinical diagnostic problem, is, in reality, quite complex. Varying combinations of the preceding conditions in a well-nourished woman can easily lead even the most thorough physician astray. It takes more effort to unravel the "toxemia syndrome" by differential diagnosis than it does to make a snap judgment.

Knowledge that malnutrition is responsible for the onset of MTLP and assiduous efforts to see that all mothers are well nourished does not mean that swelling, weight gain, protein in the urine, hypertension or convulsions and coma are going to disappear from the childbearing population. It does guarantee that mothers who are truly well nourished will not display these signs and symptoms due to MTLP.

The mother should keep in mind through all this that when she maintains a good diet her chances of developing MTLP are reduced to zero. She is also doing everything possible to reduce to the absolute minimum the chances that she or her baby will suffer any other complication of pregnancy or labor.

8

OTHER PREGNANCY COMPLICATIONS:
safeguarding mother and baby

Every expectant mother wants to enjoy her pregnancy and give birth at term to a healthy baby. A good diet is the best insurance that she will.

In addition to safeguarding the mother and baby from MTLP, a good diet offers protection from many other common complications of pregnancy. Half a century of medical and nutritional research has proved that poor diets during pregnancy cause mothers to experience more anemias, infections, placental malfunction, difficult labors, Caesarean sections, poor postpartum healing and failures at breast-feeding.

Effects of poor diet on the baby run the spectrum from prematurity and low birth weight to brain damage and stillbirth. Most of this difficulty is *preventable* through sound maternal nutrition every day throughout gestation.

Common anemias of pregnancy are primarily nutritional in origin. Most women take vitamin-mineral supplements with iron during pregnancy to maintain their red blood cell counts. If a mother shows signs of anemia, additional iron tablets are often prescribed. However, several other substances in addition to iron must be available at the same time for the manufacture of red blood cells. Chief among these is protein. Also important are folic acid, vitamin B-12, cobalt, copper and other trace elements. There may be others of which we are as yet unaware.

The best policy to follow with regard to nutrition during pregnancy is to eat a well-balanced diet each day from a wide variety of nutritious foods. In this way, protein needs are met in addition to providing other nutrients which may not yet have been recognized as important to health. The vitamin-mineral supplement is not harmful, but it cannot substitute for eating enough good foods. The mother who follows a good diet will protect herself from becoming anemic.

Late in pregnancy, many women show low red cell counts not related to true anemia. In the well-nourished woman who has not been restricting salt, the plasma volume expands dramatically. This means that her normal number of red blood cells has been diluted in the plasma so that, in a given amount of blood sampled, it appears there are fewer red cells than normal. The total number of red cells in the circulation may be actually increased. After delivery, these mothers have red cell counts that are normal since the extra fluid retained in the bloodstream during pregnancy has been mobilized and excreted.

Although anemia is generally seen to be nutritional in origin, the relationship between nutrition and severe infection remains somewhat less well acknowledged in our country despite scholarly volumes on the subject published in recent years.

The most exhaustive of these works, a World Health Organization monograph entitled *Interactions of Nutrition and Infection,* appeared in 1968. The authors are Dr. Nevin S. Scrimshaw, Professor of Nutrition and Head of the Department of Nutrition and Food Science at the Massachusetts Institute of Technology, Dr. Carl E. Taylor of the Johns Hopkins University School of Hygiene and Public Health and Dr. John E. Gordon, Emeritus Professor of Preventive Medicine and Epidemiology at Harvard. At the end of their work is a bibliography of 1,445 references to support their conclusions.

The authors show that common infections are more likely to develop into serious ones among the malnourished. In addition, infection can put stress on the body so that borderline nutritional deficiencies degenerate into severe malnutrition.

Scrimshaw and his collaborators point out that malnutrition allows certain bacteria and other germs to enter the body through the skin, respiratory tract and intestinal tract. Because the natural defense mechanisms in the poorly nourished person do not work well, once these infectious agents enter the body, they multiply at a rapid rate. Impaired by malnutrition are antibody responses, white-blood-cell function in combating germs, and other chemical and endocrine functions known to influence resistance to infection.

When the infection reaches the level of producing noticeable symptoms, the person's nutritional status is affected in several ways. Loss of appetite is one of the early signs of many infections. Treatments for disease may lead to more malnutrition, as when rigid diets or purgatives are prescribed. Infections can precipitate classical vitamin deficiency diseases such as scurvy, beriberi, pellagra and anemias due to deficiency of any of the elements necessary for building blood.

The well-nourished mother who gets a minor infection usually throws it off quickly. Rarely would a case of flu develop into pneumonia or a urinary tract infection become a severe kidney infection with sepsis. Even if the well-nourished pregnant woman should develop hepatitis due to a virus, she usually recovers without life-threatening problems.

Infections which are speedily overcome by the well-nourished woman's defense mechanisms are often severe and even fatal in the poorly nourished. Reports from India and Israel confirm that poorly nourished pregnant women have low resistance to liver infections; these disorders are a leading cause of maternal death in all the world's poverty areas. A pregnant woman who develops a liver infection is at greater risk because of the extra stress pregnancy imposes on this organ.

The liver is the master gland of nutrition. All food substances absorbed from the stomach and intestines pass directly into the liver where they are changed in various ways to provide all the cells of the body with food materials for growth, repair and energy. Special proteins, such as the albumin discussed previously, are continually formed and released into the bloodstream.

During pregnancy there is an increased need for these special proteins. Growth and development of the baby, growth of the womb, growth of the placenta, expansion of blood volume and storage of protein for use in later breast-feeding, all demand increased liver metabolism. A good diet throughout pregnancy provides the liver with the needed food substances to fulfill its round-the-clock task of cellular nutrition.

A second function the liver performs at higher levels in pregnancy is neutralizing and excreting harmful poisons which originate in the lower bowel. Termed its detoxication function, it has led to the liver being termed "the watchdog of the abdomen." All blood draining the stomach and intestinal tract goes first into the liver where it is filtered before passing into the general circulation. The liver then excretes the toxic substances in the bile and urine.

Female hormones produced in large quantities by the placenta are also detoxified and excreted by the liver. Toward the end of pregnancy, the amount of hormones produced daily is several hundred times greater than the amount contained in a birth control pill. If the mother is malnourished, the liver may fall behind in its task of clearing these hormones from the body. They then accumulate in the liver and body tissues. The well-nourished mother has a liver which can work at peak efficiency in detoxication, thus protecting herself and her baby from needless infection and MTLP.

There are other compelling reasons why the expectant mother should let nothing stand between her and good nutrition. The most feared difficulties, those which come about in labor, delivery and the postpartum period, are also related to poor nutrition.

Many women have been told that if they gain too much weight during pregnancy they will have a difficult labor and delivery. They fear being too fat by the time labor begins. They fear their baby will be too large. They fear their labor will be long and painful. They fear they will need a Caesarean section. They fear they will hemorrhage.

A look at the facts reassures the well-nourished woman. When mothers have a physiologic weight gain from eating the correct foods, very few gain excessive amounts of weight. In over 7,000 pregnancies in the Contra Costa County project, a weight gain of thirty to forty pounds was average. These mothers usually returned to their pre-pregnancy weight within six weeks after delivery. In twins, weight gains of fifty to sixty pounds are typical, reflecting, as we have seen, the greater needs of two developing babies and the marked physiologic water retention caused by the extra hormones from two placentas.

If the mother has been obese before pregnancy and switches to a higher quality diet, she may actually lose a few pounds over the course of pregnancy and, after delivery, be in much better health than previously. The focus is on adequate nutrition, not pounds. Since many American women fear gaining weight because they have been so conditioned to fear "losing their figures," it is necessary to remind them that they must gain *enough* weight during pregnancy from eating good foods. This is especially important for mothers who are underweight at conception. In fact, the only reason women should be weighed at prenatal visits is to insure they are gaining enough. When the pregnancy weight gain is the result of a sound diet, including adequate salt intake, the mother does not gain excessively, although she may gain significantly more than the old twenty-four-pound limit. One factor accounting for the larger gain is the increased amount of water retained when the mother salts her food to taste. This may add fifteen or more pounds to the mother's original weight and, usually within a week, these extra pounds vanish. Since the expanded blood volume of pregnancy required to service the placenta is no longer needed after the baby's birth, the kidneys respond by allowing the excess water to leave the body in the urine. This period of increased urination due to mobilization of fluid is called postpartum diuresis. The same nutritional factors which provide optimum conditions for maternal health during pregnancy and the growth and development of the baby also account for the physiologic weight gain in the well-nourished mother. The cultural obsession with the idea that "thin is beautiful" should be replaced, especially in the case of the expectant mother, with the concept that "health is beautiful." Not only will the healthy mother be less likely to have difficulty during pregnancy and more likely to have a larger baby who is easier to handle, but she recuperates from childbirth much quicker, too.

The works of Ebbs (1941), Burke (1943), and Higgins (1976) support the view that sound diet, increased weight gain, and larger infants do not increase the rate of obstetrical complications. In fact, they found that complications of labor and delivery are much more likely to occur among women with poor diets and underweight babies.

Dr. John Ebbs of Toronto compared the obstetrical outcomes

in three groups of mothers. One group contained 120 women whose diets were deficient and who were not counseled about nutrition in any way. The second group of 170 mothers on supposedly adequate diets received nutrition education which stressed the importance of high-quality proteins, vitamins and minerals. Ninety women whose diets were judged deficient received food supplementation in addition to nutrition education.

Difficult, slow and painful labor (dystocia) was observed in 24.2 percent of women on poor diets, compared to 2.3 percent in the supplemented group. The duration of labor and length of postpartum recovery was longest in the poor diet group. Labor averaged five hours shorter in the good diet groups. Overall, the rate of major complications reached 36 percent in the poor diet group, 12 percent in the adequate group and 9 percent among supplemented mothers.

Dr. Ebbs concluded in 1942:

> During the whole course of pregnancy the mothers on a good or supplemented diet enjoyed better health, had fewer complications and proved to be better obstetrical risks than those left on poor diets.

It should be obvious to contemporary researchers that there is no justification for pregnant women being "left on poor diets" in any sort of experimental situation. The aim of their work should be to insure that every mother has a diet adequate for pregnancy.

Bertha Burke, a public health nutritionist at Harvard, demonstrated that sound nutrition prevented many labor and delivery complications, especially MTLP. She reported in 1943 that MTLP never occurred in mothers who consumed at least 68 grams of protein daily. In contrast, 44 percent of mothers on a poor diet developed it. Overall, major delivery complications were 50 percent higher among malnourished mothers than among the well nourished.

Both Ebbs and Burke, working in the 1940's, had no institutionalized low-calorie, low-salt diet regimens or diuretic therapies to counter. However, neither one was an obstetrician, so their clinical observations made little impact on routine prenatal care or on priorities for further confirming research.

More recently, Agnes Higgins of the Montreal Diet Dispensary analyzed the obstetrical outcomes of 1,736 births to mothers in the Dispensary nutrition program. In 1,250 cases the mothers also received food supplementation. She found, contrary to general belief, that mothers with larger babies did better than those with smaller infants. Her mothers, most of whom come from low-income groups, generally gave birth to larger infants than the other patients delivering at the Royal Victoria Hospital, public and private alike. Dispensary mothers had a higher incidence of spontaneous births and a lower incidence of Caesarean sections than all other patients.

What accounts for the easier labors and deliveries of mothers with good diets? Probably most significant is the optimal growth of the uterus made possible by sound nutrition.

When a woman is not pregnant, her uterus is a small, almost solid organ about half the size of her fist and weighing only two ounces. By the end of pregnancy, it has increased in size thirty-fold to accommodate the baby, placenta, membranes and over a quart of amniotic fluid. Several changes occur to produce this striking growth. New muscle fibers are formed early in pregnancy, existing muscle fibers lengthen and enlarge and new connective tissue, collagen, is built up between muscle groups to strengthen the uterine wall. Two important nutrients fostering this process of uterine growth are proteins and vitamin C.

When adequate nutrients are not supplied by the mother's diet, the uterus does not grow normally. During labor, it is more prone to exhaustion by the strong contractions necessary to deliver the infant. When this happens, the mother may receive drugs to stimulate the uterus into further contractions or, if labor has failed to progress for some time, a Caesarean section may become necessary.

Among doctors who use good nutrition as the foundation of their prenatal care, the Caesarean section rate is approximately three percent. Depending on geographic area, this is four to ten times less than currently reported in the general population.

Among the three percent who must have a Caesarean section for some unavoidable reason, most commonly when the baby is found to be in some unusual position during labor or the mother's pelvis is too small, the well-nourished woman is still ahead. She has few problems with healing of the abdominal and uterine incisions made to deliver the baby surgically. In a poorly nourished mother, the abdominal wound may burst open a few days after delivery and have to be restitched, or the uterine scar may be so weak that it ruptures in subsequent pregnancies. It is these cases which have given rise to the adage, "Once a section, always a section." The well-nourished woman with an adequate pelvis may be able to have a vaginal delivery with a subsequent pregnancy, depending on the reason for her first section. Her uterine and abdominal scars will have healed strongly and should be able to withstand the stress of normal labor.

Most American women who give birth in the hospital undergo another surgical procedure, even when they push their babies out spontaneously without assistance from the doctor's forceps. They receive an episiotomy, or incision in the vaginal outlet, to permit the baby's head to emerge more quickly. In the well-nourished mother, the episiotomy wound heals without difficulty after the initial swelling and soreness that accompany any surgical wound.

A final difficulty related to poor nutrition which has profound effect on the newborn baby is failure of the mother at breast-feeding. Though not technically a pregnancy complication, breast-feeding often develops into a serious postpartum problem for American mothers.

Much has been published by organizations which promote breast-feeding about how to establish successful lactation. Great emphasis is placed on the importance of a nutritious diet for the nursing mother, yet nowhere is there criticism of the low-calorie, low-salt pregnancy diets and diuretics which undermine the breast-feeding efforts of so many women.

What effect do restrictive pregnancy diets have on mothers who plan to breast-feed?

In talking with women, the same story unfolds time after time: their milk "dried up" a few days after they returned home from the hospital. Generally, these women are disbelieved and their failures attributed to their "not really wanting to nurse in the first place" or "being too lazy to take the time" or "just being too nervous." Overlooked is the fact that the mother who has cut down her salt intake, her calorie intake and her protein intake during pregnancy is unlikely to have enough stored fluid, fat and protein to sustain a good milk flow. Effectively, the mother has been "dried up" before she even begins breast-feeding.

Paradoxically, her baby also suffers dehydration at birth and will require more fluid in the early days of life to counteract the effect of the diuretics. This baby demands more from the mother who has least to give. Bottle supplementation with commercial formula is the usual prescription from pediatricians who are also unaware of the effects of the restrictive pregnancy diets. With less stimulation from the baby's suckling, the breasts produce even less milk. Breast-feeding becomes a token proposition or, more often, is wistfully terminated a few days after birth.

Both mother and baby lose when breast-feeding fails. Apart from the well-documented psychological advantages to mother and baby, breast-feeding provides each with incomparable physical benefits as well.

The uterus must stay tightly contracted in the days after birth in order to prevent excessive bleeding from the site where the placenta was implanted during pregnancy. When the mother nurses her baby, a natural hormone is released which causes efficient uterine contractions. The mother who does not breast-feed runs a higher risk of postpartum hemorrhage due to uterine relaxation.

Research on the nutritional value of human milk supports what breast-feeding mothers have known all along: breast milk is best milk. The proteins in human milk are utilized almost 100 percent by the baby's immature digestive system, reducing the chances for stomach upset or colic in the newborn. Mata and Gyorgy reported in a symposium sponsored by the American Society for Clinical Nutrition that breast milk also contains immunological properties which can never be duplicated by any type of artificial formula. The early milk, colostrum, is especially high in these factors which are effective against an astonishing array of organisms responsible for the bulk of common pediatric disorders—and frantic calls to the pediatrician's office from new mothers! Diarrhea, salmonella, staph and strep infections, allergic reactions, Coxsackie virus, shigella, polio and respiratory infections are all markedly less common in breast-fed infants. Every mother who desires the best start for herself and her baby will begin nursing as soon after the birth as possible, ideally on the delivery table or in the recovery room, but certainly within the first four hours. Thereafter, babies should be nursed on demand. This assures that the mother's milk will come in within a day or two at most so that the baby will not lose more than a few ounces in the early days of life. In all these ways breast-feeding smoothes the postpartum course for mother and baby.

The mother who follows a sound diet every day of gestation protects herself from common obstetrical complications. Moreover, she also protects her baby from the most ominous of newborn problems, low birth weight.

9

THE AFFLICTED CHILD:
preventing low birth weight

More than 240,000 low-birth-weight babies are born annually in the United States. The percentage of such babies has risen steadily since the early 1950's. By 1968, 7.7 percent of all American babies were underweight at birth according to government sources. If a spring 1976 survey of four thousand new mothers done by *Mothers' Manual* is reliable, the figure has skyrocketed to 13.5 percent among middle and upper income families.

The 1972 United Nations Statistical Handbook discloses that low birth weight runs up to 60 percent higher in the United States than in some other advanced nations. The figures for Scandinavian countries show they have reduced low birth weight to 3 percent. In the People's Republic of China, it is less than 3 percent.

What is going wrong?

Does a baby's birth weight matter that much?

Definitely. Birth weight is the most accurate indicator of a baby's health and future mental and physical development. Babies born underweight have markedly reduced chances for survival, for normal intelligence and for coordinated movement. A report by the U.S. Department of Health, Education and Welfare in 1972 detailed the higher risks of death and permanent disability faced by the underweight newborn. Two-thirds of all deaths occurring up to the twenty-eighth day of life happen to low-birth-weight babies. This death rate is thirty times higher than in babies of normal birth weight.

Half of all low-birth-weight babies will grow up with I.Q.'s of less than 70, the cutoff point for severe mental retardation.

Three and a half times more infants of low birth weight suffer other neurologic deficits, such as cerebral palsy, epilepsy, learning disabilities and behavioral disorders.

It is a grim picture. Yet low birth weight does not arise from unknown cause. It is not a matter of heredity. In fact, the vast majority of cases are completely preventable. Every mother can take steps to protect her unborn baby from low birth weight by following a good diet during pregnancy.

It has been known since the 1920's that maternal nutrition influences birth weight more than any other factor. Many international researchers and practitioners have long since proved that the quality of the mother's diet has everything to do with her baby's birth weight and subsequent development.

A landmark volume presenting the writings of just a few standouts would include:

Honora Acosta-Sison, Philippines, 1929
Guttorum Toverud, Norway, 1931
Sir Edward Mellanby, England, 1933
Winslow T. Tompkins, 1941
John Ebbs, Toronto, 1942
Bertha Burke, Boston, 1943
A. N. Antonov, Russia, 1947
William Dieckmann, Chicago, 1951
Reginald Hamlin, Australia, 1952
Hilda Knobloch and Benjamin Pasamanick, New York, 1956

   Benjamin Platt, England, 1964
   Thomas Brewer, San Francisco, 1966
   Leela Iyengar, India, 1967
   J. F. Kerr Grieve, Scotland, 1974
   Agnes Higgins, Montreal, 1976

Jay Hodin, executive director of the Society for the Protection of the Unborn through Nutrition (SPUN) and author of an exhaustive analysis of studies on malnutrition and developmental disabilities, has noted: "Many of these investigators report results in which the probability that prenatal nutrition is unrelated to infant health is *less than one in a billion.*"

In most of their papers one finds appeals for aggressive action to prevent low birth weight. The prescription, based on their own clinical experience, is almost always the same: improve maternal health by dietary intervention and low birth weight will virtually disappear.

Just what constitutes low birth weight? What size baby is normal? For many years, the figure five and a half pounds was used as a line of demarcation between low and normal birth weight. This figure was also used as the official standard for determination of prematurity. Most of these cases of low birth weight traditionally have been accounted for by a shortened period of gestation, with less than the thirty-eight weeks considered the minimum time necessary for complete fetal development.

In recent years, however, there had been a dramatic upsurge of low-birth-weight at term babies—those who weigh less than five and a half pounds after a full forty weeks gestation. There is evidence that these babies are at far greater risk than those born too early. The concept of "weight for gestational age" is replacing the straight five and a half pounds as an indicator of a baby's chances for normal health and development. Under this system, the underweight-for-date baby causes more concern among high-risk nursery personnel than the infant who is premature, but normal-weight-for-date. Both types of low-birth-weight infants result primarily from maternal malnutrition.

Agnes Higgins of Montreal has stated that any baby weighing less than seven pounds at birth reflects some degree of sub-optimal maternal nutrition. Many agree with her that five and a half pounds may be a valid indicator for infant survival, but mere survival is not enough, especially when it is possible with our present knowledge and resources to feed every pregnant woman the diet she and her baby need for optimal health. Mrs. Higgins, whose program at the Montreal Diet Dispensary includes distribution of milk, eggs and oranges to women who need them to supplement their diets, pegs the cost of this extra food at $125 per pregnancy. The cost of maintaining a low-birth-weight baby in an intensive care unit can exceed $300 a day. The cost of institutionalizing a severely retarded child for life runs to $900,000.

Following the lead of Bertha Burke with whom she studied, Mrs. Higgins stresses a high-protein, high-calorie diet: she aims for 100 grams of high-quality protein and 2,600 calories a day. Mothers with twins require an additional 30 grams of protein and 500 extra calories—all provided by an extra quart of milk daily.

Burke found that the level of protein intake in the diet is directly reflected in the length and weight of the child at birth. In her 1940's study groups at Harvard, all babies weighed at least six pounds when the mother's diet contained 80 or more grams of protein a day. The median weight in this group was eight and a half pounds. When mothers obtained less than 45 grams of protein daily, 47 percent of the babies weighed under five and a half pounds.

Burke determined that for every additional 10 grams of protein added to the mother's diet (up to 100 grams), the baby's
birth weight would increase by one-half pound. Iyengar in India
substantiated that this could be done as late as the last four weeks
of gestation with positive effect on the baby's birth weight.

How exactly does the mother's diet determine the way her baby
grows? As we have mentioned, the placenta is the organ which
nourishes the baby from the earliest weeks of pregnancy. A multi-
service organ, it works as the baby's stomach, liver, kidneys, and
lungs until the moment of birth. At birth, a healthy placenta
weighs one and a half to two pounds, is the size and shape of a
small dinner plate and is an inch or more thick. Its large flat surface is firmly attached to the wall of the uterus where, under normal conditions, it remains throughout labor, separating from the
uterus and being expelled only after the baby is born. Blood vessels form a network throughout the placenta, feeding into the
baby via the umbilical cord. The cord is the lifeline from mother
to baby through which 300 quarts of blood per day are circulated.
Many square yards of contact surface develop in the placenta
over the course of pregnancy to facilitate the vital exchange of
nutrients and waste products between mother and baby.

After the mother eats a meal, the food is digested, absorbed,
and passed into her liver which then releases essential nutrients
into her bloodstream. These predigested nutrients reach a level of
concentration higher in the mother's blood than in the baby's, so
they readily pass through the very thin walls of the baby's capillar-
ies into the baby's circulation. This process of diffusion works the
same way in the transfer of oxygen from mother to baby. The
nutrient-rich blood finally circulates through the baby's liver where
the nutrients are recombined into the protein building blocks the
baby needs for growth and development. There is no direct mix-

ing of the baby's blood with the mother's. Each remains in its own circulation. Yet, they are intimately connected.

The outdated idea that the placenta can somehow extract nutrients from the mother which are not in her circulation is a threat to sound pregnancy nutrition. In a sense, the baby is in competition with all the tissues of the mother's body which also require continual nourishment from her bloodstream. If the mother fails to take in all the essential nutrients in large enough proportions to sustain the increased demands of pregnancy, her baby will not magically receive what it needs for optimal growth. The baby does not have top priority for nutrients. In fact, there are numerous reliable studies which show the opposite.

Aaron Lechtig and his collaborators have reported that even moderate maternal malnutrition interferes with the process of placental cell proliferation, resulting in abnormally small placentas. When the size of the placenta is reduced, the surface area available for nutrient transfer is correspondingly reduced. Many researchers now conclude that small placentas result in low-birth-weight babies. Very simply, a small placenta cannot transfer as many nutrients to the growing baby as a larger one. So, the baby does not weigh as much as it should at birth, even if it is born at term.

During the last eight weeks of pregnancy the baby gains an ounce a day. Brain development is occurring at the most rapid rate ever. The baby requires more oxygen and nutrients of all types—including proteins, vitamins, minerals and calories—than earlier in pregnancy. If the mother is told she has gained enough weight already and put on a low-calorie, low-salt diet at this crucial time, the baby will be denied the nutrients needed to accomplish normal development. A restrictive diet is also likely to cause the mother's blood volume to shrink, reducing the amount of blood flowing through the placenta. The baby can suffer intrauterine growth retardation from this reduction of placental blood flow. When less blood passes through the placenta, fewer nutrients pass to the baby during any given period of time.

The *National Institutes of Health Collaborative Study of Cerebral Palsy* in 1968 drew a clearcut relationship between weight of the placenta and birth weight of the baby. When the placentas in one study group weighed only seven to fourteen ounces, over 22 percent of the babies weighed less than five and a half pounds. In another group, the placentas weighed fourteen to twenty-one ounces and low birth weight dropped to 3 percent. In over 1,700 cases the placenta weighed more than twenty-one ounces. Low birth weight fell to 0.5 percent in this group! A total of 31,966 infants were evaluated in this study, a large enough sample to meet any standard of scientific evidence! Clearly, maternal nutrition governs the size of both placenta and baby. It is also responsible for the secure implantation of the placenta on the uterine wall.

Abruption of the placenta (its premature separation from the wall of the uterus before the baby is born) is one of the most lethal complications in obstetrics. Traumatic abruption is the unfortunate result of an accident in which the mother suffers puncture wounds to the abdomen. This freak occurrence could happen to anyone, well nourished or not. Typically, however, abruption is a severe manifestation of malnutrition. Seen most frequently among the poor, medical literature reports case after case of recurrent abruptions in the same mother. Abruption often accompanies underlying metabolic disease, such as MTLP.

Any degree of abruption is an immediate hazard to the baby's survival. Once the placenta has separated, no oxygen can be transferred to the baby. Toxic wastes soon build up in the baby's tissues. The brain can only survive eight minutes of oxygen deprivation without irreversible damage. Roughly 50 percent of babies die before mothers with this complication can reach the hospital. Immediate delivery is the only treatment. An attempt is made to save the baby, if possible, at the same time attention is being given to minimize the internal blood loss and resulting shock which can kill the mother, too.

Nontraumatic abruptions do not occur in well-nourished women. Good nutrition early in pregnancy fosters secure implantation of the placenta on the uterine wall. Continued good nutrition assures that the placenta will grow to meet the demands of the developing baby.

In the last trimester, a healthy placenta is necessary for optimal development of another crucial organ, the baby's brain. The brain grows in two ways. Cells divide to make new ones and individual cells enlarge as they mature. Malnutrition retards both these processes, but it is especially devastating during the period when new cells are forming.

Cell division is most rapid and, therefore, most vulnerable from one month before birth until five months after. Never again will the baby's brain experience such an incredible proliferation of new cells. All of the eleven billion neurons, the cells which process and analyze information, are formed before birth. Inadequate nutrition during gestation results in permanent, irreversible deficits in the number of cells which make up the baby's brain.

Other problems also arise. Without adequate nutrition, the brain cells which do exist are likely to be malformed and their interconnections impaired. Learning problems and poor motor coordination are traced by many pediatric neurologists to these abnormalities.

Dr. Arnold Gold of Columbia University, addressing the Fall 1976 meeting of the American Foundation for Maternal and Child Health, stated his belief that minimal brain damage in all social groups is primarily the result of intrauterine malnutrition. In his own practice he sees children who have a variety of difficulties which he attributes in many cases to minimal brain damage not readily discernible at birth. Their parents or teachers report the children are hyperactive, have a short attention span, are frustrated easily, are delayed in meeting developmental milestones, have poor coordination and poor school performance or seem immature.

Citing the work of Knobloch and Pasamanick who in the 1950's outlined a "continuum of reproductive casualty" caused by low birth weight, Dr. Gold charted the overt and minimal damage done to cerebral function by malnutrition:

FUNCTION	OVERT	MINIMAL
MOTOR	Cerebral palsy	Clumsiness
SENSORY	Blindness	Impaired spatial
	Deafness	perception and
		shape memory
MENTAL	Low I.Q.	Poor abstract
		reasoning
		Hyperkinesis
SPEECH	Aphasia	Delayed speech
		Language difficulties
CONVULSIVE	Epilepsy	Abnormal electro-
		encephalogram (EEG)

Very little maternal malnutrition is required to produce these abnormalities. Researchers in England, for example, think even mild degrees of maternal undernutrition in the last few weeks of gestation can compromise the intricate process of brain cell division and integration. Especially vulnerable in their view is the cerebellum, the part of the brain which coordinates voluntary muscular movement.

Dr. Benjamin S. Platt, of the London School of Tropical Medicine, produced these disorders experimentally by restricting protein and calories in pregnant animals during his 30 years of research. He believed that the consequences of protein-calorie malnutrition which he documented in over five thousand laboratory cases were the same in human mothers as in other species of mammals. A member of the World Health Organization Joint Expert Committee on Nutrition for many years, Platt wrote that his colleagues treated his thesis with "undisguised scorn . . . because of the tendency, particularly marked among clinicians, to ignore or disparage experimental work on animals, often for no other reason than because the results have been obtained on animals."

Platt summarized his findings in 1968:

> We have found throughout our experimental work that the earlier in life the animal is subjected to dietary deficiency, the more pronounced and extensive are its effects. . . . Malnutrition lowers maternal efficiency and leads to the production of underweight babies, many of whom will die before reaching two years of age, whilst among their survivors there will be some who never reach their full physical or mental potential. . . . Expert committees have met to discuss the problem of "low birth weight," though, still, I may say, with scant attention to the possible role of the nutrition of the mother.

When physicians responsible for giving prenatal care discount the work done on nutrition in animals, they are left with few guidelines for human nutrition. Doctors who treat the malnutrition thesis of reproductive casualty with "undisguised scorn" often state that they would be convinced if somebody would show them results of a truly controlled experiment in which some mothers were starved and others fed. To obtain the results to satisfy them, human mothers, pre-selected to share characteristics of statistical significance, would have to spend their entire pregnancies in a laboratory. Their diets would be rigidly managed so no deviations would be possible. Their rates of exercise, rest and sleep would be recorded, along with notations of how much of each food each mother ate. Mothers' weight gains and losses would be charted. Fetal and placental growth and maturation would be determined by a sophisticated battery of tests. All mothers would be monitored, as were the astronauts in space, twenty-four hours a day.

After the babies were born they would be wired for metabolic assessment, too. A computer might have to be installed to handle all the information about differences between deprived and well-fed infants.

The researchers would then spend five years converting all their data to mathematical models, publishing their formulas, addressing major scientific symposia and establishing their academic reputations as unbiased investigators of the most impeccable order.

In fact, it will never be possible to satisfy the demands of those who call for inhumane experimentation of this sort. So, these physicians will continue to remain unconvinced of the evidence that speaks for the importance of their pregnant patients' nutrition. They will continue to promote the view that "There's no hard data proving that nutrition has anything to do with pregnancy outcome" —a classic Catch-22.

History, however, has provided analogous situations in which human mothers, albeit not pre-selected, have been subjected to severe nutritional deprivation on a large scale. These historical "experiments" support the malnutrition thesis and discredit other theories which have obscured its role for many years.

The most stark example comes from the World War II Nazi blockade of Leningrad. During the seventeen-month siege, from August 1941 to December 1942, no food could be shipped into the city. The conditions of famine were so harsh than many women ceased menstruating, few conceived, and among those who did, the rates of spontaneous abortion, stillbirth, infant mortality and low birth weight surged upward.

A. N. Antonov, a Russian pediatrician who lived and worked through the siege, reported his observations in one clinic in the *Journal of Pediatrics* in 1947. One of the most striking developments he noted was the drastic decline in births (despite the fact that much of the army had retreated into the city). From 3,867 in 1941 the number plummeted to 493 in 1942. Of these, 414 occurred in the first half of the year—babies conceived before the siege began. Only 79 were born in the second half of 1942—those conceived after the siege began.

The 414 babies born in the first half of 1942 were subjected to severe intrauterine malnutrition during the last half of pregnancy, the critical period of brain development and weight gain. Of them, 49 percent weighed less than five and a half pounds at birth. Forty-one percent failed to attain normal length, measuring less than eighteen and a half inches. In the first half of the year, 256 of the 414 died—an infant mortality rate of 618 per thousand. Antonov described the babies as being frail with thin skull bones and high-pitched cries. They sucked poorly on mothers who produced little milk.

Dr. Antonov concluded:

> Hunger, vitamin deficiency, cold, excessive physical strain, lack of rest, and constant nervous tension had their effect on the health of the women, and the intrauterine development of the fetuses, and the condition of the newborn children during the siege . . .
>
> The cause of the unusually high proportions of premature births and of stillbirths in the first half of 1942 was hunger during pregnancy, that is, the insufficient quantity and unsatisfactory quality of the women's food.

In addition to these catastrophic effects on the unborn, maternal starvation was also responsible for a five-fold increase in convulsive MTLP, reported later by Persianov, a Moscow OB/GYN specialist.

What does this tragic story from the past have to do with American obstetrics today? The message is clear: mothers must not be starved during pregnancy and though most American women may not literally be hungry, those who receive inadequate and incorrect advice about their diets are starving for the nutrients they and their babies need.

At the top of the list of malnourished pregnant women are those who have been told by their doctors to:

1. restrict weight
2. restrict salt
3. take diuretics

Virtually every pregnant woman in America in the last thirty years has been exposed to one or another of these useless pieces of dietary advice at some point in her pregnancy, which accounts for the widespread upsurge of low birth weight and brain-damaged children in our country. As Dr. Arthur Sackler, international publisher of the *Medical Tribune*, commented in 1974:

> I don't know how much more one needs to shock our medical consciences. One does not have to be a physician to be concerned with the epidemic of defective neonates (babies less than twenty-eight days old). . . . Nothing can be lost and potentially infinite suffering may be prevented by instituting simple, preventive nutritional measures and withholding questionable medications during pregnancy.

Dr. Charles Lowe, then scientific director of the National Institute of Child Health and Human Development, agreed in 1972 after reviewing the dramatic decline in low-birth-weight rate (from

13.7 percent to 2.8 percent in women having their first babies) in the Contra Costa County prenatal clinics during the toxemia prevention project. Recognizing that this result was obtained exclusively by the use of scientific nutrition education and the abandonment of symptomatic therapies, Dr. Lowe commented:

> These conclusions challenge the conventional wisdom, which demands constraint on weight gain by caloric restriction, a limitation of salt intake, and the use of saline diuretics. None of these were used in the Brewer series. . . . Why is our prematurity rate rising, a factor of life in no other advanced nation? The answer may well lie in our prenatal regimens. It looks as if we can make real progress on both questions merely by feeding pregnant women.

All these conclusions point to the fact that we already have a reliable method for the prevention of many of the common complications of pregnancy, in particular of the metabolic toxemia of late pregnancy and of low-birth-weight babies. It is clearly improper to say that we need "more studies" before implementing sound maternal nutrition for all pregnant women. To continue to study the ravages of these preventable complications in pregnant women and their babies is to cruelly ignore the evidence already available.

Obstetricians trained in the United States over the past twenty years will probably continue to have trouble accepting the "new look" in human maternal-fetal nutrition. Each one will only be able to learn for himself by trying these methods with pregnant mothers. As with all other stages in their training, they will have to learn by doing. As they do, they will be gratified by the healthful outcomes produced by this approach to pregnancy management.

10

"WHAT MEDICAL SCHOOL DID YOU GRADUATE FROM?":
the doctor's training excludes nutrition

The mother who begins to question the wisdom of her doctor's diet and drug practices can act on the nutrition information she has and keep quiet about what she's doing. Or, she can attempt to persuade the doctor that there is merit in her ideas.

Mothers who choose the second course should be prepared for confrontation. Depending on his degree of tolerance for lay opinions, the physician's attitude toward a mother who tries to raise the issue of pregnancy nutrition may range from disagreeing to patronizing to hostile.

Sooner or later, the doctor who resents such attempts at continuing education from a patient will try to terminate the conversation with a question he knows to be irrelevant: "What medical school did you graduate from?" That medical school is the only repository of valuable information is a misconception commonly held by physicians. In fact, mothers should understand that junior-high-school home economics courses probably teach more about applied human nutrition than the doctor has learned in his entire professional life. She has missed nothing in this area by not being a medical school graduate.

What does a mother need to know about her doctor's training in order to place his nutrition advice into proper perspective?

A review of the applied nutrition education programs provided by American medical schools leads one to conclude that knowledge of pregnancy nutrition is considered completely unnecessary for the trained obstetrician.

Not one U.S. medical school requires that every student study applied human nutrition in order to receive the M.D. degree.

Not one department of obstetrics/gynecology requires that residents know and apply the principles of scientific nutrition as part of their specialty training.

Not one professional medical organization, the American Medical Association (AMA) and the American College of Obstetricians and Gynecologists (ACOG) included, has adopted official standards for managing pregnancy nutrition.

Not one local, state or federal health agency has such standards.

Standards have been established which mandate tests for syphilis, rubella, Rh incompatibility and anemia on every pregnant woman, yet nothing is done to require evaluation of her nutrition—even though far more mothers and babies are at risk because of malnutrition than all the other factors combined.

Several characteristics of OB/GYN training help explain how neglect of pregnancy nutrition has become institutionalized in our country. Most important, the emphasis in an OB/GYN residency is on learning how and when to do operations. Because the goal is to produce skilled practitioners who can perform life-saving, complicated surgical procedures under the most adverse conditions, scant attention is paid to *preventing* the conditions which cause some of these dire problems. Gynecological surgery, because of its "interesting" surgical complexities—especially when cancer is involved—is in the forefront of most residents' minds. Each resident must carry out a specified number of each type of operation in order to meet the minimum requirements of the specialty. With residency requirements so skewed in the direction of technical competence in the operating room, it is not surprising that interest in pregnancy nutrition is virtually nil. Malnutrition cannot be corrected surgically.

In this training program, one waits for disease to occur, then valiantly struggles to restore some semblance of health to the patient. With few exceptions, the OB/GYN resident learns to view himself as an expert in the treatment of disease, rather than in the preservation of health. Scant attention is paid to what amounts to 90 percent of the obstetrician's routine practice—the birth of normal babies to healthy mothers. There is little study of the conditions that produce normality. A "normal" is rarely presented as a case worthy of study as senior physicians make rounds, quizzing residents as they go. As Frank Hytten has observed in his text, *Physiology of Pregnancy,* it has only been in the past twenty years that any interest in the events of normal pregnancy has been shown by those in academic medicine. As it stands now, the health concerns of 90 percent of childbearing women are not being addressed in disease-oriented OB/GYN residencies. At the accustomed rate of change in medical practice, it will be another fifty years before preventive measures are given the same amount of attention now devoted to salvage efforts.

Another difficulty arises from the prevalent attitude that if the professor didn't say it or do it, it's not important. An unquestioned line of authority governs the transmission of information and attitudes within the apprentice-system of physician training. Doctors seem to have great difficulty making changes in their practices because often no one in authority mandates them. Because nutrition is a relatively new science and medicine one of the oldest, few medical school professors know of the work which has been done in the field. Those who do not know cannot teach. *Optional* lecture courses on nutrition do not adequately reflect the importance of the subject in maintaining health. There is no quicker way to convey the impression that something is unimportant than to make it optional!

Increased specialization within the whole health care field has resulted in the isolation of the OB/GYN resident from other specialists and professionals from whom he could learn much about preventive prenatal care. The pediatrician's training should include constant interaction with the obstetrician, yet the tendency has been for the obstetrician to focus on the mother and let the pediatrician care for the baby after it is born. Even when prenatal regimens ordered by the obstetrician have proved damaging to the unborn baby, the pediatrician has been unwilling to suggest changes. Instead, a new, glamorous subspecialty has emerged in the last decade in pediatrics—perinatology. It delivers intensive care to sick, primarily underweight, newborns, another addition to the world of "rescue" medicine.

An impasse results when professional training programs become so narrowly focused that they provide nutrition information, but no medical background, for nutritionists and a glut of pathology, but no nutrition education, for physicians. Worse yet, doctors who are ignorant of the protective benefits of sound prenatal nutrition tend to lack respect for the work of nutritionists. This observation could also be made with regard to nurses, physical therapists, laboratory technicians and public health workers. Many physicians seem to have the attitude that these highly skilled people are menials whose only responsibility is to carry out the physician's orders.

It is ironic that the professional with the least competence in the field, the obstetrician, wields absolute authority over the pregnancy nutrition of his patients. At best, he views nutrition counseling as something apart from the scientific prenatal care he gives—an optional frill done by somebody else down the hall. At worst, he considers it not at all—often leaving the mother to follow a drug company diet sheet he routinely distributes to patients.

The epidemic of "high-risk" mothers and defective infants spawned by the adoption of low-salt, low-calorie diets and diuretics in the United States has curiously elevated the status of obstetricians, not lowered it. Commanding sophisticated hardware born of space-age technology, the obstetrician is being counted on to aggressively manage every pregnancy and labor with increasing emphasis on intervention. Amniocentesis, sonar, oxytocin challenge tests, external and internal fetal monitoring, fetal scalp blood sampling during labor, and the inevitable soaring rates of Caesarean section are the current answers to a problem which should never have materialized. Instead of asking *why* the epidemic exists, American obstetricians have plunged in to "rescue" the casualties —all in the best tradition of crisis medicine. "Regionalization" of perinatal health care is being urged since small community hospitals cannot afford to maintain the costly intensive care maternity and neonatal units now considered to be the hallmarks of quality obstetrical care. In the process, efforts to establish standards for scientific nutrition management in pregnancy stagnate.

A final consideration is the way OB/GYN physicians come to think about the women they see in their practices. Most medical training reinforces the idea that mothers, or any non-doctors, for that matter, cannot possibly assume responsibility for any aspect of their medical care. Quite simply, the common assumption is that it is too difficult for the average person to understand; therefore, the obstetrician doesn't need to try to share his knowledge with his patients. Many women complain about the paternalistic way their questions are handled by their obstetricians. Too often, the response boils down to: "Don't worry your pretty head over such matters. I'll take care of it just fine." The role of the doctor has not included a teaching function, except within the confines of medical school where knowledge is passed on to others deemed suitable for admission to the medical fraternity. The authoritarian tradition in obstetrical training has bred a generation of doctors many of whom are unprepared to deal with the increasingly better-educated women they serve in private practice. In the clinic situation, disparity in social and economic class between doctor and mother aggravates the problem. There is probably nothing further removed from the inclination and training of the obstetrician than sitting down with a mother in the clinic to discuss her diet.

Since the doctor's OB/GYN training excludes consideration of nutrition, every mother needs to know how to manage this aspect of her own pregnancy. The subject is not complicated. It originates in the mother's kitchen, in her food planning and in her control over what she purchases for herself and her family. She does not require a prescription or a laboratory experiment to intelligently handle the weekly marketing.

11

FOODS FOR LIFE:
a clinically proven pregnancy diet

Nutrition science over the past fifty years has clearly defined what constitutes a good, balanced diet for pregnancy. Yet, whether an American mother and her unborn baby are adequately nourished continues to be a matter of luck, not science.

For most American women pregnancy may be the first time in their lives they give serious thought to their nutrition—*if the subject is brought to their attention*. When the mother knows that her baby's future health and mental development are at stake, she refuses to take chances with her diet. She seeks the best possible foods she can afford. She is not concerned with the bare minimums needed to scrape through pregnancy, though this topic seems of all-consuming interest to those who draft government nutrition standards. Her goal is giving birth to the healthiest infant possible. If this were established as governmental policy for every pregnant woman, not just those who manage to educate themselves about their needs, vast improvements in our country's maternal and infant health statistics would result.

Many women must accomplish optimum nutrition on a budget,

but it is a fallacy to assume that just because a mother has plenty of money to spend on food she is well nourished. In order to benefit from her affluence, the mother must choose, prepare and eat the correct foods, that is, those of highest nutritional value. Unfortunately, even among physicians who recognize the value of good nutrition in pregnancy, there is a tendency to assume that every woman is well nourished unless she presents some obvious sign of serious nutritional deficiency, such as anemia. Instead, the doctor must learn to regard every expectant mother he cares for as malnourished until proven otherwise. And the proof does not come until the baby has been born!

Dr. Mary Ellen Avery reported from Johns Hopkins University that up to 80 percent of the six thousand mothers she studied had insufficient protein intake during pregnancy. "Ironically," she wrote, "the women in this study were not poverty-stricken. They had enough to eat, but chose the wrong foods."

What are the correct foods for pregnancy? Very simply, the basic foods which have been the foundation of healthful diets for centuries: dairy products, meat, seafood, fruits and vegetables, nuts and seeds, grains, salt and water. Eating well for pregnancy does not mean cutting out foods, but rather being sure to include enough foods from all the nutrient groups. For many, "going on a diet" for pregnancy will mean eating more, not less, than before while enjoying a wider variety of foods. This diet is one which emphasizes the pleasure as well as the healthfulness of good eating!

This is the same diet plan developed for the successful Contra Costa County toxemia prevention project. It is simply the U.S. Department of Agriculture's "basic four" adapted to the special needs of pregnant women. As charted below, the daily food plan groups foods according to their nutritional makeup. Key foods in each group are listed as superior sources of specific nutrients.

110

PREGNANCY DIET CHART

FOOD GROUP	MINIMUM NUMBER OF SERVINGS PER DAY	SOURCES
MILK	4 glasses (one quart)	whole, skim, low fat, buttermilk, powdered, evaporated, yoghurt or cheese may be substituted. See Protein Counter for equivalents.
EGGS	2	may be fixed any style, used in recipes
MEAT, FISH, POULTRY, MIXED VEGETABLE PROTEINS, CHEESE, NUTS	2	See Protein Counter for complete lists of these foods.
DARK GREEN LEAFY VEGETABLES	1 large or 2 medium	beet, collard, dandelion, mustard or turnip greens, kale, Swiss chard, spinach, lettuce, cabbage, escarole, endive, broccoli
WHOLE GRAINS, BREADS, CEREALS	5	whole-grain flours, oatmeal, 100% bran flakes, Wheatena, shredded wheat, wheat germ, granola, corn bread, corn tortillas, corn or bran or whole-wheat

PREGNANCY DIET CHART

FOOD GROUP	MINIMUM NUMBER OF SERVINGS PER DAY	SOURCES
		muffins and rolls, waffles, brown rice, whole grain pancakes, El Molino, puffed cereals
VITAMIN C FOODS	2—either piece of fruit or large glass of juice	whole potato (any style), large green pepper, grapefruit half, whole orange, lemon, lime, papaya or tomato, cantaloupe, strawberries, parsley
FATS	3 tablespoons	butter, vitamin A enriched margarine, oils
YELLOW OR ORANGE FRUITS, VEGETABLES	5 per week	apricots, cantaloupe, cherries, papaya, peaches, prunes, tangerines, oranges, watermelon, corn, pimientos, squash, sweet potatoes, tomatoes, wax beans
LIVER OR KIDNEY	once a week	beef, calf, chicken
SALT	to taste	
WATER	to thirst	

The overall aim is for the mother to have 2,600 calories and 100 grams of protein each day, plus all the salt and other essential minerals and vitamins she needs. To simplify matters, quantities are expressed in servings. A look at the Protein Counter at the end of the book gives an idea of typical serving sizes. In normal pregnancy, the mother develops a good appetite, so the single rule governing amounts of food is: eat to appetite.

Mothers who are underweight at conception may have much larger appetites than those of normal weight. Mothers expecting twins, as we have discussed, need a minimum of 500 more calories and 30 grams more protein daily. One extra quart of milk each day satisfies these needs, but the mother may meet them by eating more of other high-protein foods if she prefers.

A quart of milk and two eggs a day form the foundation of this diet *for every pregnant woman*.

These foods provide high-quality, complete protein, they contain all other known vitamins and minerals in forms the body assimilates easily; and they are comparatively inexpensive as sources of high-quality nutrition—the best buys in the market in terms of food value per dollar spent. Though milk and eggs are balanced foods designed by nature for the sustenance of life, both have come under attack as contributors to ill health!

Some people worry about eating too many eggs because of the widespread publicity about their high cholesterol content. Many of these "cholesterol information" commercials seen daily on television are sponsored by companies who market "egg substitutes," and these advertisements fail to mention certain important facts: cholesterol is manufactured by the body independent of dietary intake. Also, experts in coronary disease are divided over whether it is excess cholesterol in the diet or a defect in the cholesterol manufacturing mechanism which produces a cholesterol build-up which can lead to heart attack. More important, it makes no difference to the pregnant woman who is right about cholesterol build-up. Some researchers believe that women in the childbearing years are protected from heart attack by their female hormones. The incidence of heart attack in women begins to rise after menopause, when their circulating hormone levels fall. Many other dietary and social factors affect the cholesterol level in the blood. Sugar and refined flour consumption are both associated with elevated cholesterol levels, for instance. Blaming heart attacks on eggs alone is really a very simplistic concept.

About one in three people don't eat eggs for another reason: they don't like them. Pregnant women in this group must come to look on eggs as medicine—a big pill—because of their nutrition. However, they needn't be gagged down plain. Recipes using them in eggnog, French toast, creamed soups and sauces, casseroles, puddings and other desserts follow in the meal plans.

The current disenchantment with milk stems from certain theories of academic nutritionists who lack clinical experience. First, there are supposed to be large numbers of people, primarily Blacks, who cannot tolerate milk because they are reputed to lack an enzyme, lactase, which permits their bodies to metabolize lactose, the sugar in milk. This lactase deficiency theoretically produces severe cramps, nausea and diarrhea whenever milk is ingested. While this metabolic problem may indeed afflict a small number of people who made up the study groups for the researchers forwarding this thesis, Tom rarely encountered—in daily practice among a clinic population that was comprised of 50 percent Black patients—an individual who was truly allergic to milk. When someone did report such a problem, it was just as likely to be a white as a Black patient. He found when counseling pregnant women, regardless of their race, the question to ask was, "Can you drink milk?," not, "Do you like milk?" The answer to the first was almost always "Yes"; to the second, often "No."

The pernicious effect of the "lactase deficiency" theory has been to influence clinic nutritionists across the country to stop recommending milk as a basic food for Black mothers. Many of these nutritionists think it cruel to even suggest that these mothers drink milk. Instead of seeing "lactase deficiency" as the rare condition it is, the idea that "Blacks can't drink milk" has passed into general acceptance, thus robbing low-income Black mothers of an inexpensive, high-protein, vitamin- and mineral-rich food.

A second objection to milk for pregnant women comes from those who are still worried about a mother's sodium intake. As with most high-protein foods, milk does contain a good deal of sodium. But, as we have seen, excess sodium is efficiently excreted by the kidneys so there can be no retention of dangerous levels of the mineral in the body. Women need more salt when they are pregnant and milk is an excellent source.

The final concern about milk—whole milk in particular—is that it is fattening. Whole milk does contain more butterfat than skim, and therefore more calories per glass, but whole milk meets the needs of pregnant women better than any other type, in part because it does have extra calories. The calories provided by fat are important in pregnancy to spare protein for use in building the baby's body and brain. The fat in whole milk also is present in the correct amount to promote the most efficient absorption of calcium by the body. Calcium is needed in much higher quantities throughout pregnancy to help grow strong teeth and bones in the developing baby. The primary teeth begin to form during the fifth month of gestation and the baby's skeleton begins to change from cartilage to bone early in the sixth month. These processes are seriously undermined when the mother's diet is low in calcium. Furthermore, if her diet supplies plenty of calcium, but not enough fat, the calcium will not be assimilated. Sometimes in cooking, another type of milk, skim, low-fat, powdered or evaporated, may be called for, but as a rule whole milk is preferable. As far as protein is concerned, the values for the different types of milk are exactly the same, eight grams per eight ounces.

For those who dislike the taste of milk, there are many forms of it other than as a beverage. Yoghurt, cheese and ice cream all are substitutes which, incidentally, are usually well tolerated by those with a true milk allergy. The Protein Counter indicates how much of each is the protein equivalent of a glass of milk.

In addition to sodium and calcium, milk contains other minerals and all vitamins except C. The other foods on this diet build on the complete nutrition foundation provided by milk and eggs.

Three of the most important vitamins for a pregnant woman are A, C and folic acid (part of the B complex). Vitamin A has been called the ("anti-infection" vitamin since the 1930's. Mothers who have a balanced diet with adequate vitamin A seldom develop serious infections of the kidneys, bladder, uterus, lungs, liver or breast during pregnancy or after delivery. In malnourished women, on the other hand, such life-threatening infections are common. Vitamin A keeps skin healthy and helps the lining of the female tract, bladder, kidneys, stomach, intestines and bronchial tree resist infection by bacteria. Foods containing vitamin A, in addition to whole milk and eggs, are the yellow and orange fruits and vegetables and the dark, green leafy vegetables. There is vitamin A in butter and margarine. Most vitamin capsules also provide vitamin A. It is best to obtain nutrients from foods, but taking a vitamin and mineral supplement daily is additional insurance against a deficiency. Of course, such supplements do not provide protein, calories or salt, so they must not be relied on for complete nutrition.

Vitamin C is exceptionally important. It helps the uterus grow strong, and so makes for an easier labor and birth. Poorly nourished women have thin, flabby wombs which function poorly and result in longer labor. Sometimes the uterus is so weak it ruptures during labor—even with a very small baby. In addition to the citrus fruits, vitamin C is found in many other foods. Strawberries, cantaloupes, tomatoes, broccoli, cabbage, green peppers and potatoes also supply considerable amounts.

Folic acid is part of the complex of nutrients needed to build red blood cells. Iron, protein and vitamin B12 are also part of this complex. The best sources of these nutrients are liver and kidney, eggs, and dark green leafy vegetables. Liver may be ground and used as a spread for snacks or put into a loaf with other ground meat. Liverwurst is a more nutritious choice for a lunch meat than bologna. Since folic acid is water soluble, cooking greens and throwing away the water, as most people do, results in loss of this vitamin. Using these vegetables in salads is far better. Raw spinach, especially for those who dislike it cooked, makes a delicious addition to or substitute for lettuce.

Eating these vegetables raw is the beginning of another healthful habit—processing food as little as possible in order to conserve nutrients. Raw fruits and vegetables of all kinds provide fiber for the digestive system, an important consideration for pregnant women who are often troubled with constipation as the uterus enlarges and displaces the intestines. For the same reason, whole grains—in breads, cereals, and baked goods—are much more healthful than white bread or flour.

Whole grains are whole because they contain the entire kernel as it grows in nature, including the bran and the germ, both of which are stripped in the refining process. The bran provides fiber and B vitamins, the germ is high in vitamin E. Bread and cereal manufacturers make a token attempt to replace these nutrients, adding back eight of the 22 removed, then calling their products "enriched." Breads and cereals are also significant in the pregnancy diet because they furnish calories from carbohydrates to spare protein and provide energy. Nuts and nut butters, particularly the old standby, peanut butter, are excellent foods, too. They are high in protein, vitamin E and energy calories from fats.

To accompany solid foods at mealtimes, or alone as snacks, fresh fruit and vegetable juices, milk and broth or bouillon are far superior to coffee, tea, soda, juice "drinks" and "punches." These no-nutrient beverages should be sharply limited during pregnancy. They are expensive and a real impediment to good nutrition when they replace natural juices in the diet. Coffee, tea and most soft drinks contain caffeine, a substance which over-stimulates the glands which regulate blood sugar. Over-consumption of these drinks results in a metabolism which runs at top speed for a brief period, then "crashes" when the excess sugar is removed from the circulation. Mothers who rely on these beverages to satisfy their thirst and fill their stomachs between meals are subverting their own nutritional interests.

The same is true of mothers who smoke instead of eat during pregnancy. Much publicity has been given to the notion that smoking in and of itself causes low-birth-weight babies. Only when the mother uses cigarettes as a substitute for good food does she run the risk of having a sickly baby. None of the studies on smoking in pregnancy has compared the nutrition of the mothers as a variable influencing birth weight of babies in the study group. Yet, it is a truism that when people give up cigarettes, they begin to eat more.

Of course, it is a good idea to stop smoking at any time of life because cigarettes cause so many debilitating diseases. They also cost money which might better be spent on good food. If stopping completely seems impossible, cutting back to a few cigarettes a day is still beneficial. Doing away with cigarettes usually rejuvenates the taste buds, so the mother who hasn't had a good appetite in pregnancy may suddenly experience a renewed interest in eating.

Other situations over which the mother has less control may also adversely affect her appetite—even when she has the correct information about nutrition and the means to obtain it. The most common one is the nausea and vomiting or heartburn many women at times experience in pregnancy. A related problem is the "too full" feeling of late pregnancy when it is uncomfortable to eat a complete meal. The best way of coping with these situations is to eat small meals throughout the day, "grazing" as it were, instead of sitting down to three large meals. It helps to eat protein, especially during the night when the mother has to get up to urinate. Having a glass of milk, a hard-boiled egg, a slice of cheese or meat, or a cup of yoghurt helps keep the mother's blood sugar up around the clock. A protein feeding during the night helps prevent that weak feeling in the morning which can bring on nausea. So-called "morning sickness" usually goes away in a few weeks, but if the mother actually vomits after eating, she should try to keep up with her nutrition by eating again as soon as possible. In severe cases, she may require medication to control the vomiting. There is a tendency in a busy obstetrics practice for the doctor to brush aside this complaint simply because it is so common and because most physicians have not been trained to be vigilant in safeguarding the mother's nutrition. Because prolonged vomiting can threaten the mother's entire metabolism, it must be accorded importance by the physician and treated swiftly.

Nutrition awareness should make the prospective mother a very tough customer when she shops for food. First in her shopping cart are those foods she knows she needs for a healthy pregnancy and normal baby. She spends much more time at the fresh produce counter than in the canned vegetable section. The meat and poultry department wins out over the TV dinners. Rolled oats, nuts and raisins are taken home to be mixed into granola while sugar-loaded imitations are left on the shelves. This mother knows that every procedure done for her by someone in a food processing plant adds to the final purchase price of each item. So, she chooses to buy the basic foods in their most natural form and prepare them simply at home.

What an old fashioned idea! Yet it not only conserves nutrients, it saves money as well. One stunning example: a fourteen-cent pound of peeled, sliced, raw potatoes costs $1.41 when purchased as potato chips. A ten-fold increase!

The few extra minutes it may take a mother to carefully choose from the basic foods is made up when she completely bypasses those aisles crammed with garish displays of nutritionally bankrupt foods: soft drinks, snack foods, candy, commercial cakes, cookies and pastries, boxed cereals, white bread, dessert mixes, soup mixes, salad dressing mixes, bread and roll mixes, drink mixes, prepared breakfasts, prepared lunches, prepared dinners—all left behind. What a sense of triumph, a feeling of power, to breeze by these devitalized substitutes for real food! What a pleasure to find that the basic foods save money and build health for every member of the family!

A fine guide to this form of nutritionally alert shopping is Nikki and David Goldbeck's 1973 paperback, *The Supermarket Handbook: Access to Whole Foods*. They guide the shopper through each section of the market, telling in great detail how to determine quality and freshness in every type of food. When possible, they recommend, by brand name, some prepared foods that, in a pinch, can substitute for homemade. Their main criteria for food selection are the products' freedom from additives and sugar.

One hundred five pounds of sugar per year per person is consumed in the United States. That works out to five hundred totally empty calories every day, calories the pregnant woman should be getting from nutritious foods. Sugar does not build a baby's body or brain! The additives, ten indiscriminately mixed pounds of them per person per year in the United States, are potential causes of birth defects. They have never been tested for their effects on the unborn baby, so it is best to avoid them during pregnancy.

Happily, any mother can remove herself and her unborn baby from the category of experimental animals by deciding to rely on the basic foods, prepared at home, for family meals. For women who were lucky enough to grow up in families where home cooking was the rule, respect for food preparation is handed down from mother to daughter. Years of helping stir the sauce, knead the dough and grate the cheese are cultural inheritances priceless in today's fast-food society. When she has a kitchen of her own to run, she sees cooking as a creative, loving enterprise—not a chore to be greeted with the same amount of enthusiasm usually reserved for taking out the garbage. She welcomes the opportunity to prepare good food for her loved ones, knowing she is shaping their health for years to come.

The late Adelle Davis, a pioneer in bringing nutritional awareness to millions of people, wrote:

> The health of yourself and your family is a mirror which reflects your intelligence, your efficiency and your cooking methods. If you purchase your foods wisely, plan your menus carefully, prepare meals with minimum nutritive loss . . . then you, your children and your husband can probably possess as vibrant and buoyant health as it is possible for good nutrition to give.
>
> To the mother of such a family come pride of accomplish-

ment and deep satisfaction of a job well done. She has shouldered her tasks and seen to it that good health has come from good cooking.

The menus and recipes in the following chapters are designed with the nutrition-conscious, pregnant cook in mind. The menus are formulated to meet or surpass, on a daily basis, her pregnancy nutrition requirements. Recipes feature a protein-per-serving notation. In this way, the mother who wishes to experiment with her own menus will find it easy to keep track of her daily protein intake. She need only remember to take in eighty to one hundred grams of protein a day. As long as the daily food plan is followed, the foods may be combined in any manner that suits the cook and her family!

For those who wish to create their own recipes or see how family favorites rate nutritionally, a Protein Counter lists basic foods, the amount of protein in a given amount of edible food (excluding skin, bones, peelings, etc.), and the source of the protein—either animal or vegetable. Since vegetable proteins are incomplete, that is, lacking some of the essential building blocks (amino acids) which make them completely usable by the body, it is wise to include protein from animal sources at the same meal or in the same recipe with vegetable proteins. Some familiar combinations are chili con carne or macaroni and cheese. Protein from animal sources, in these cases, meat and cheese, is complete and boosts the nutritive value of the vegetable proteins, the beans and noodles, it accompanies.

Ellen Buchman Ewald and Frances Moore Lappé have written extensively on combining vegetable and dairy proteins as a way of increasing the protein content of vegetarian diets. Their books contain information about protein complementarity and should be consulted by mothers who follow vegetarian diets.

Absolute vegetarians who use no animal protein in their diets must be extremely careful in planning their pregnancy diets. The Seventh Day Adventist Church provides information on total vegetarianism as it is part of their religious practice. A wiser course is to suspend absolute vegetarian diets during pregnancy and nursing. At the very least, they should be modified to include eggs and milk products. An absolute vegetarian diet which may sustain a nonpregnant woman will not suffice for pregnancy. For the sake of her baby, the sensible mother will obtain all the high quality, complete protein she needs regardless of its source.

12

MENUS FOR LIFE:
sample menus for pregnancy

DAY 1

BREAKFAST
* Tropical Oranges
  Fried eggs
  Sausage links
  Raisin toast
  Milk

LUNCH
* Cream of Tomato Soup
  Grilled cheese sandwich
* Green Bean Salad
  Iced tea

SNACK
Salted nuts
Cantaloupe wedge

DINNER
* Salad Niçoise
* Bouillabaisse
  Garlic bread

DESSERT
* Cream Puff
  Milk

* See next chapter for this recipe. Recipes are indexed beginning on page 215.

DAY 2

BREAKFAST
* Ambrosia
* High-Protein Pancakes
  Maple syrup, butter
  Milk

LUNCH
* Coleslaw Deluxe
* Tuna Roma
  Milk

SNACK
Banana filled with peanut
butter
Milk

DINNER
* Nancy's Eggplant Salad
  Baked Potato
* Broccoli Parmesan
  Roast chicken
* Real Lemonade

DESSERT
* Broiled Peach Amandine
  Milk

DAY 3

BREAKFAST
* Stewed Prunes with Cashews
* Cheese Omelet
  Cornbread

LUNCH
* Tomato Salad with Basil
  Raw green pepper stuffed with
    chicken salad
* Whole-Wheat Bun
  Milk

SNACK
* High-Protein Brownies
  Milk

DINNER
  Escarole salad
* Oil and Vinegar Dressing
* Cream of Mushroom Soup
  Baked sweet potato
  Roast loin of pork, sliced

DESSERT
* Baked Apple, Bonne Femme
  Milk

DAY 4

BREAKFAST
* Apricots in Honey Cream
  Poached eggs
* Bran Muffins
  Milk

LUNCH
* Cream of Asparagus Soup
  Lamb shish kebab
  Middle East flat bread
  Lemon tea

SNACK
* Charlotte's Gazpacho
  Cheese and crackers

DINNER
  Molded vegetable salad
  Egg noodles
  Green peas, buttered
  Swiss steak
  Milk

DESSERT
* Coconut Pudding

DAY 5

BREAKFAST
* Bananas Baltimore
* High-Protein Granola
  Milk or yoghurt

LUNCH
Marinated mushrooms
* Italian Sweet Sausage in
  Pastry
* Mustard Sauce
  Minestrone soup

SNACK
Raw vegetable platter
Deviled egg halves

DINNER
Tossed green salad
* Roquefort Dressing
* Corn Chowder
  Sautéed liver
  Fried onions and bacon

DESSERT
* Fresh Fruit Tart
  Milk

DAY 6

BREAKFAST
* French Strawberry Pancakes
* Orange Sauce
  Ham slice
  Milk

LUNCH
* French Onion Soup
* Chef Salad
* Reuben Sandwich
  Milk

SNACK
* Cheese popcorn
  Cranberry juice

DINNER
* Antipasto
* Lasagna
  Italian bread

DESSERT
Chocolate pudding
Espresso coffee

DAY 7

BREAKFAST
* Citrus Punch
  Apple crisp
  Sausage patties
  Milk

LUNCH
* Avocado-Grapefruit Salad
* Fish Bisque
* Cheese Polenta

SNACK
* Stuffed Dates
  Milk

DINNER
* Carrot-Raisin Salad
  Creamed spinach
* Beef Fondue
  French bread

DESSERT
* Rice Pudding

DAY 8

BREAKFAST
* Rhubarb with Pineapple Sauce
  Lox
  Whole-wheat bagels
  Cream cheese

LUNCH
* Carrot Soup
  Yellow wax beans, buttered
  Corned beef hash with eggs
* Vermont Brown Bread
  Milk

SNACK
* Stuffed Celery
  Mixed vegetable juice

DINNER
* Vichyssoise
* Spinach-Orange Salad
  Corn-on-the-Cob, buttered
    and salted
* Shrimp Scampi

DESSERT
Mincemeat pie
Milk

DAY 9

BREAKFAST
Melon wedge with berries
Wheatena, cooked in milk,
 with raisins
Toast
Peanut butter

LUNCH
* Cream of Split Pea Soup
* Cheese Crackers
 Egg salad sandwich with
  lettuce and tomato

SNACK
Yoghurt with fresh fruit
Graham crackers

DINNER
 Tossed green salad
* Oil and Vinegar Dressing
 Boiled potatoes
 Boiled beets
 Corned beef and cabbage
 Milk

DESSERT
* Pumpkin Pie
 Cheddar cheese wedge

DAY 10

BREAKFAST
* Cranberry-Orange Relish
  French toast
  Bacon
  Milk

LUNCH
* Cream of Chicken Soup
  Submarine sandwich
  Potato salad

SNACK
* Liver Pâté Anderson
  Rye crackers

DINNER
* Chinese Asparagus Salad
  Cauliflower with
    * Cheese Sauce
* Crêpes Lake Forest
  Tomato juice

DESSERT
* Fruit Fondue
  Milk

DAY 11

BREAKFAST
* Grape Delight
  Poached eggs
* Blueberry Muffins
  Milk

LUNCH
* Green Pepper Salad
  Baked tomatoes
* Welsh Rarebit
  Toast points

SNACK
Canned sardines
Whole-wheat melba toast
* Mustard Sauce

DINNER
* Greek Salad
* Elsie's Pizza

DESSERT
* Egg Custard

DAY 12

BREAKFAST
Honeydew melon with
   prosciutto
Whole-wheat toast
Scrambled eggs
Milk

LUNCH
* New England Clam Chowder
* String Bean Casserole
  Bacon, lettuce and tomato
     sandwich

SNACK
Beef or chicken broth,
   bouillon or consommé
   (canned)
Croutons

DINNER
* Red Cabbage Salad
* Spinach Soufflé
* Bermuda Scallops
  Iced tea

DESSERT
* Peach Upside-Down Cake
  Milk

DAY 13

BREAKFAST
Tomato juice
Herbed omelet
Rye bread
Raspberry tea

LUNCH
* Cuban Black Beans
  Yellow summer squash,
    buttered
* Baked Cod Fillet
* Susan's Buttermilk Biscuits
  Milk

SNACK
* Peanut Butter Cookies
* Eggnog

DINNER
Swiss chard salad
* Oil and Vinegar Dressing
* Ratatouille
* Cheese Fondue
  French bread

DESSERT
* Strawberry Pie

DAY 14

BREAKFAST
* Fruit Curry
* Cheese Blintzes
  Sour cream

LUNCH
Tossed green salad
* Yoghurt Dressing
* Egg Drop Soup (Stracciatella)
* Turkey Pot Pie
  Milk

SNACK
* Egg Custard

DINNER
Marinated artichokes,
  pimientos and olives
* Spaghetti and Meatballs

DESSERT
* Espresso Ice Cream Sundae

13

RECIPES FOR LIFE:
preparing quality foods at home

The most important thing about the recipes here is not the way the ingredients are combined, but *the ingredients themselves*. From the point of view of nutrition, it makes no difference at all whether a mother eats simply or elegantly. The food value of scrambled eggs, bacon, toast and milk is the same as Quiche Lorraine! The only difference is in the way the dishes look when the preparation is complete, and, of course, for those who enjoy cooking, the adventure of making something special from simple ingredients.

All these recipes have been "pregnancy-tested"—with excellent results. Many of the Italian dishes I remember watching my grandmother prepare on holidays or vacation days when I would visit her farm in central New York. Others have been developed over the years. A few are delicious contributions from friends.

A major goal is to encourage mothers to try cooking from scratch instead of relying so heavily on the prepared and processed foods so readily available to us. When food is prepared at home, the cook knows exactly what's in it! And what isn't. The mother who gets into the habit of cooking from the basics is also much less likely to feed her baby prepared baby food, of compromised nutritional value.

In the interests of the best nutrition, no sugar or white flour is used in the recipes. Except for the very rare item that just doesn't taste right unless made *exactly* as mother did (Christmas cookies, for instance), we now use honey and whole wheat flour.

Other general principles include:

1. Use fresh vegetables and fruits whenever possible, frozen otherwise. Canned goods have been overcooked, which causes a loss of nutrients and texture.

2. Buy bacon, sausage, hot dogs, lunchmeat, ham only if product is free from nitrates and nitrites. It is possible to find these in the supermarket, or to request of the manager that they be stocked in the frozen food sections. Nitrates and nitrites are used as preservatives. They are known to be cancer-producing, and are absolutely un-needed in foods which can be preserved perfectly by freezing. If there is a store nearby that features unprocessed foods (sometimes called a "natural" or "health" food store) it usually has such products, but often at incredibly inflated prices.

3. Buy breads and pasta made from whole grains or make them at home; Buitoni noodles and some Pepperidge Farm and Arnold Bakery breads are exclusively whole-grain, though they may contain sugar or corn syrups. Again, ask your store manager to stock these brands if you don't see them on the shelves. Store loaves of bread in the freezer. That way you don't have to worry about mold-inhibitors, dough conditioners and flavor enhancers, and other unnecessary preservatives.

Dishes listed in the Menus chapter, but not found here, can be found in any good cookbook. Our favorites are:

Nourishing Your Unborn Child, Phyllis Williams, R.N. (New York: Avon, 1975)

Features in-depth discussion of various nutrients and their functions in the body and many natural food recipes for pregnancy.

Menus for Entertaining, James Beard (New York: Delacorte, 1965)

Inventive and dashing food combinations with excellent instructions on preparation methods.

Foods of the World series (New York: Time-Life)

Fascinating tours of the world's cuisine, beautifully illustrated and easy-to-follow directions.

The Vegetarian Epicure, Anna Thomas (New York: Knopf, 1972)

Delicious no-meat cookery, including menus.

The Cheese Book, Vivienne Marquis and Patricia Haskell (New York: Simon & Schuster, 1965)

All about the world's cheeses and how to use them in cooking.

A World of Breads, Dolores Casella (New York: David White, 1966)

All sorts of breads, rolls, muffins, pastries, pancakes, waffles, coffee cakes, and specialty breads from all over the world, 600 recipes.

The Vermont Year Round Cookbook, Louise Andrews Kent (Boston: Houghton Mifflin, 1965)

A homey, talky cookbook that takes you into the writer's kitchen as well as through the seasons; fine section on tools, terms and tips.

The Rodale Cookbook, Nancy Albright (Emmaus, Pa.: Rodale Press, 1973)

A bible for organic food preparation.

Joy of Cooking, Irma Rombauer and Marion Becker (Indianapolis, Ind.: Bobbs-Merrill, 1975)

A bible for traditional food preparation, with vast stores of information about food selection as well.

The recipes are arranged by the food groups they stress. Happy eating!

I.
Eggs, Milk and Cheese

CHEESE BLINTZES

MAKES: 12 filled pieces
PROTEIN: 8 grams per piece

Batter

> *3 eggs, at room temperature*
> *1 cup milk*
> *1 teaspoon vanilla*
> *2 tablespoons honey*
> *1 tablespoon corn oil*
> *¼ teaspoon salt*
> *1 teaspoon baking powder*
> *¾ cup whole-wheat flour*
> *Butter*

Beat eggs lightly in a bowl. Add milk, vanilla, honey and oil. Sift salt, baking powder and flour into liquid mixture and stir just until flour lumps dissolve.

Drop by the tablespoon onto a 6-inch buttered hot skillet or

crêpe pan and tilt pan so that batter spreads evenly over the
bottom. Cook over medium heat until light brown, then turn and
cook briefly on other side just to dry surface. Stack blintzes until
ready for filling.

Filling

> 1½ cups cottage cheese, preferably small curd
> 2 eggs
> 3 tablespoons orange juice concentrate
> ¼ teaspoon salt
> 2 tablespoons honey
> ½ teaspoon cinnamon

Preheat oven to 425°.

Blend all ingredients thoroughly in a bowl. Place 2 tablespoons
of filling in center of the darker side of each blintz. Roll into tube
shape and turn ends under to seal.

Arrange filled blintzes in a single layer in a buttered glass baking dish; brush tops with melted butter. Bake for 15 minutes, or
until golden brown. Serve hot with sour cream.

CHEESE CRACKERS

MAKES: 5 dozen 2-inch crackers
PROTEIN: 2 grams per cracker

> 2 cups sharp Cheddar cheese, grated
> 5 eggs, beaten
> ½ cup powdered milk
> 2 teaspoons celery salt
> 1 teaspoon garlic powder
> 1 teaspoon Worcestershire sauce
> 2 teaspoons paprika
> 1½ cups whole-wheat or rye flour
> ¾ cup soy flour
> ¾ cup wheat germ
> ¼ cup poppy seeds
> ⅓ cup corn oil

Preheat oven to 400°.

In large bowl, combine cheese, eggs, milk and seasonings. Stir thoroughly so that all milk powder is moistened. Add flours, wheat germ, seeds and oil. If necessary, a small amount of water may be added to form a stiff paste.

Roll out on floured surface to a thickness of ¼ inch. Cut into 2-inch squares and bake on an ungreased baking sheet for 10 minutes, or until lightly browned.

Serve warm with soups, dips or as snacks.

CHEESE FONDUE

MAKES: 4 servings
PROTEIN: 35 grams per serving

> 1¼ cups dry white wine
> ¼ teaspoon garlic powder
> 1 pound Swiss cheese, grated
> 1 teaspoon cornstarch
> Salt and pepper to taste
> 2 loaves whole-wheat French bread, in 2-inch cubes

Pour the wine into a fondue pot or medium-sized saucepan and heat over medium heat until small bubbles rise to the surface. Do not boil. Add garlic powder, then cheese ¼ cup at a time, stirring continually. Allow each portion of cheese to dissolve completely before adding more. Dissolve cornstarch in 2 teaspoons water and add. When mixture begins to bubble, add salt and pepper to taste and place serving pot on table over a warming candle or hot tray.

Each person spears the bread chunks with a sharp-tined fork and swirls them around in fondue mixture until coated. Keep fondue at even temperature, just bubbling, to avoid cheese forming a ball. If mixture becomes too thick, stir in a little warm wine.

CHEESE OMELET

MAKES: 2 servings
PROTEIN: 19 grams per serving

> 4 eggs
> ¼ cup hot water
> ½ cup Cheddar cheese, grated
> 2 tablespoons butter

Beat eggs thoroughly in a bowl. Add water and mix well. Melt butter in a skillet and pour in egg mixture. Cook over medium heat. As eggs start to firm, gently lift up edges with spatula, tilting pan so that remaining liquid can seep underneath and cook. When eggs resemble a soft pancake, sprinkle cheese on top, then fold whole omelet in half. Bottom should be golden brown and center creamy. Cut in two pieces and serve at once.

To vary, omit cheese and use instead:

> *2 tablespoons onions, diced*
> *½ teaspoon sage*
> *¼ cup parsley, chopped*
> *3 tablespoons sour cream*

CHEESE POLENTA

MAKES: 8 servings
PROTEIN: 25 grams per serving

> *6 cups milk*
> *4 tablespoons butter*
> *3 cups yellow cornmeal*
> *1 teaspoon salt*
> *3 eggs, beaten*
> *1 cup mozzarella cheese, grated*
> *¾ cup Parmesan cheese, grated*

Preheat oven to 375°. Oil an 8- by 13-inch shallow baking pan.
Heat milk and butter in a large saucepan until butter melts. Stir in cornmeal and salt and cook over medium heat stirring continually, for about 15 minutes, or until mixture thickens enough

to hold spoon erect. Add eggs and cheese and mix thoroughly. Mixture should be somewhat dry.

Spoon mixture into pan and bake approximately 45 minutes. When done, polenta will be lightly browned and knife inserted into center will come out clean.

Let cool in pan until polenta can be cut into squares. Serve warm or cold.

COCONUT PUDDING

MAKES: 4 cups
PROTEIN: 21 grams per cup

> *1 cup powdered milk*
> *⅓ cup clover honey*
> *¼ teaspoon salt*
> *4 whole eggs*
> *2 egg yolks*
> *3 cups milk*
> *1 tablespoon vanilla*
> *2 tablespoons cornstarch*
> *2 cups shredded coconut*

In a large saucepan, combine powdered milk, honey and salt. Add eggs and yolks and 1 cup of the milk. Stir until the powdered milk is dissolved and eggs are thoroughly mixed. Beat until smooth with an electric mixer. Add remaining milk and vanilla and bring to boiling point over medium heat.

In separate cup, put 4 tablespoons of the mixture and add cornstarch. Stir until cornstarch is completely dissolved, add to the contents of the large saucepan and stir for 1 minute.

Remove from heat and mix in shredded coconut.

Pour into serving dish, let cool to room temperature, then chill. Serve sprinkled with toasted coconut or semi-sweet chocolate slivers.

To vary, substitute 1½ cups sliced bananas for coconut, or substitute ⅓ cup cocoa for coconut and boost honey to ½ cup. Both of these variations make excellent pie fillings.

CREAM OF ASPARAGUS SOUP

MAKES: 4 bowls
PROTEIN: 11 grams per bowl

> *1 pound fresh or frozen asparagus*
> *2½ cups chicken broth*
> *½ cup onion, chopped*
> *½ cup celery, chopped*
> *1 large potato, thinly sliced*
> *2 cups milk*
> *3 tablespoons butter*
> *2 hard-boiled eggs, sliced*

Rinse fresh asparagus, then cut off tips and place them in a basket to be steamed over the other ingredients as they simmer.

Cut asparagus stalks into pieces and place them in a large saucepan with the chicken broth, onion, celery and potato. Bring to a boil, then reduce heat and insert steamer basket with asparagus tips above liquid. Cover all and simmer for 25 minutes, or until soft.

In a separate saucepan, heat the milk and butter until butter melts.

Set steamer basket aside and beat cooked broth with an electric mixer until smooth, or pour 1 cup at a time into blender, cover and blend for a few seconds at high speed. Then return to large saucepan.

Add hot milk and butter to vegetable mixture and stir thoroughly. Garnish with asparagus tips and egg slices. Serve hot.

CREAM OF CHICKEN SOUP

MAKES: 4 bowls
PROTEIN: 16 grams per bowl

> 1½ cups (6 ounces) cooked chicken, diced
> 2½ cups chicken broth
> 1 cup onion, chopped
> ½ cup parsley, chopped
> 1 large potato, thinly sliced
> 2 teaspoons salt
> 2 cups milk
> 3 tablespoons butter

Place all ingredients except milk and butter in a large saucepan. Bring to a boil, then reduce heat and simmer covered for 20 minutes, stirring occasionally.

Blend with an electric mixer or blender until smooth. Add milk and butter and stir thoroughly while bringing just to boiling point. Serve hot, garnished with parsley.

To vary, add 1 teaspoon curry powder and ½ teaspoon garlic powder instead of parsley. Garnish with paprika.

CREAM OF MUSHROOM SOUP

MAKES: 4 bowls
PROTEIN: 11 grams per bowl

> ¾ pound (3 cups) fresh mushrooms, chopped
> ¾ cup onion, chopped
> 4 tablespoons butter
> 2 tablespoons whole-wheat flour
> 1 teaspoon salt
> 2 cups beef broth
> 2 cups milk
> ½ cup powdered milk
> 4 egg yolks, beaten, at room temperature
> Chives

In a saucepan, sauté mushrooms and onion in butter until onions become transparent. Stir in flour and salt, then add beef broth, milk and powdered milk. Stir until all milk powder lumps dissolve. Bring to boiling point, but do not boil.

Remove from heat and cool slightly. Stir in egg yolks. Garnish with chopped chives. Reheat and serve hot.

CREAM OF SPLIT PEA SOUP

MAKES: 4 bowls
PROTEIN: 14 grams per bowl

> *3-inch cube salt pork*
> *1 cup dry split peas*
> *1 cup fresh or frozen peas*
> *¾ cup carrot, chopped*
> *¾ cup celery, chopped*
> *¾ cup onion, chopped*
> *1 large potato, thinly sliced*
> *1 teaspoon garlic powder*
> *1 teaspoon salt*
> *2 cups chicken broth*
> *1 cup milk*
> *Pepperoni slices*

Place all ingredients except milk and pepperoni into a saucepan. Bring to boiling point, then cover and reduce heat. Simmer 30 minutes, or until split peas are soft. Check occasionally to see that there is enough liquid to prevent scorching, and stir often. Add water if needed.

Blend until smooth with an electric mixture or blender. Add milk and bring to boiling point. Garnish with pepperoni slices and serve hot.

CREAM OF TOMATO SOUP

MAKES: 4 bowls
PROTEIN: 10 grams per bowl

> 4 tablespoons tomato paste
> 2 cups very ripe fresh tomatoes, chopped (canned whole
>   tomatoes may be substituted in winter)
> 2 cups potatoes, thinly sliced
> 2 cups onions, thinly sliced
> 2 cups beef broth
> 1 teaspoon salt
> 1 cup Cream Sauce (see page 174)
> ½ cup powdered milk
> Croutons

Place all ingredients except cream sauce, powdered milk and
croutons in a large saucepan. Bring to a boil and simmer 30 minutes, covered, until potatoes and onions are very soft.

Blend with an electric mixer or blender until smooth. If necessary, pour through a strainer to remove seeds and skin of tomatoes.
Add cream sauce and powdered milk, stirring until milk lumps
dissolve. Bring to boiling point. Garnish with croutons and
serve hot.

NOTE: This soup cannot be made with fresh tomatoes found in
the supermarket in winter. Such tomatoes are too woody in texture
and lack the succulence of those picked ripe from the vine in
summer. Most often, they have been picked green and exposed to
a gas during storage, which makes them look red though they are
not anywhere near ripe. They are a waste of money.

CREAM PUFFS

MAKES: 12 3-inch puffs
PROTEIN: 2 grams per shell; 7 grams per pudding-filled cream puff

Shell

> ⅓ cup butter
> ½ cup milk
> ⅔ cup whole-wheat flour
> ¼ teaspoon salt
> 3 eggs, at room temperature

Preheat oven to 450°.

Heat butter and milk in a medium-sized saucepan until butter melts. Add flour and salt and stir vigorously until mixture forms a ball in the center of the pan.

Remove from heat and drop in eggs, one at a time, stirring until each egg is completely absorbed and batter appears glossy, but stiff.

Drop by the tablespoon onto an oiled baking sheet. Each puff should be no larger than 3 inches across or it may not rise during baking.

Bake at 450° for 10 minutes, then reduce heat to 350° for 25 minutes. Shells should be browned and crisp when done. Open the oven door to let them cool on baking sheet before removing from oven.

To fill, cut out a circle from the top of shell with a sharp knife. Remove any threads of moist dough from inside and let stand open briefly to dry inside. Spoon filling into shell, replace top and serve. Each puff holds about ¼ cup of filling.

Fillings: Coconut or chocolate pudding, egg custard, whipped cream, ice cream, lemon pie filling, fresh fruit. For lunch, try creamed meats or vegetables—an elegant way to serve leftovers.

EGG CUSTARD

MAKES: 4 cups
PROTEIN: 17 grams per cup

> *2½ cups milk*
> *¾ cup powdered milk*
> *⅓ cup honey*
> *¼ teaspoon salt*
> *4 eggs, beaten*
> *2 egg whites*
> *1½ teaspoons vanilla*
> *Nutmeg*

Preheat oven to 325°. Oil a quart and a half shallow baking dish or casserole.

Place all ingredients into a bowl and blend until smooth with an electric mixer on low speed.

Pour mixture into the oiled dish and set it in a pan of hot water in the oven. Water should reach halfway up the sides of the dish. Bake for 50 minutes or more. Custard is done when a knife inserted near the edge comes out clean. Custard continues to cook while cooling. Cool to room temperature on rack, then chill.

Serve topped with fresh fruit.

EGG DROP SOUP (STRACCIATELLA)

MAKES: 4 bowls
PROTEIN: 8 grams per bowl

> 2 eggs
> 2 tablespoons Parmesan cheese, grated
> 2 tablespoons whole-wheat flour
> ⅛ teaspoon salt
> 3 cups chicken or beef broth
> Nutmeg or garlic powder

In a large bowl, beat eggs, Parmesan, flour and salt until smooth. Add ½ cup of broth, and a pinch of nutmeg (for chicken broth) or a pinch of garlic powder (for beef broth). Mix.

Bring remainder of broth to a boil and pour in egg mixture, beating vigorously with a fork or wire whisk. Reduce heat and simmer about 2 minutes, stirring continually, or until eggs form thready strands.

Serve hot.

EGGNOG

MAKES: 1 glass
PROTEIN: 18 grams per glass

> ¾ cup milk
> ¼ cup powdered milk
> 1 egg
> ½ teaspoon vanilla
> 1 teaspoon honey
> Nutmeg

Place all ingredients in a blender and mix for 10 seconds at high speed, or place in a small bowl and beat with electric mixer for 30 seconds.

Pour in a tall glass and sprinkle with nutmeg.

ELSIE'S PIZZA

MAKES: 2 8-slice pizzas
PROTEIN: 16 grams per slice

Dough

> 1 package dry yeast
> ¼ cup warm water
> 4 cups whole-wheat flour
> 1 teaspoon salt
> 1 tablespoon olive oil

In a cup, dissolve yeast in warm water.

Place flour and salt in a large bowl. Add yeast liquid, then slowly add water until flour gathers into a ball. Mix in oil with fingers and work until dough is elastic.

Cover with a damp kitchen towel and set in unheated oven to rise until doubled in bulk, about two hours.

Sauce

> 1 pound Italian sweet sausage, casings removed
> 1 large onion, chopped
> ½ teaspoon garlic powder
> 1 six-ounce can tomato paste
> 1 32-ounce can tomato purée
> 1 eight-ounce can mushroom pieces
> 2 bay leaves
> 2 tablespoons dried parsley

In a large skillet, brown sausage, onion and garlic powder. Remove mixture from skillet and stir tomato paste in drippings until they are absorbed.

In a large saucepan, combine tomato purée, mushrooms and seasonings. Add browned sausage mixture and tomato paste. Bring to boiling point over medium heat, then reduce heat and simmer about two hours.

Topping

> 3½ cups mozzarella cheese, shredded
> 1⅓ cup Parmesan cheese, grated
> Anchovies (optional)

Preheat oven to 400°. Pour olive oil on pizza pans.

To assemble pizza, roll out dough on floured surface to fit size of pan. Lift with both hands and transfer to pan. Pizza will recede a bit from edges of pan, floating on the oil.

Spread tomato sauce generously over dough surface. (If there is more sauce than you need, save it for pasta.) Then sprinkle cheese evenly over top. Anchovies may be used as your taste dictates.

Bake at 400° for ½ hour on bottom rack of oven.

When done, crust will be golden brown and cheese will be melted. Use a spatula to lift pizza and a large dressmaker's scissors to cut it while hot. Serve immediately.

ESPRESSO ICE CREAM SUNDAE

MAKES: 1 serving
PROTEIN: 15 grams per serving

> ⅔ cup vanilla ice cream
> ½ banana, sliced
> ½ cup peanuts, salted
> 1-ounce square semi-sweet chocolate
> ¼ cup espresso coffee, hot

In a dessert bowl, place ice cream, banana and peanuts. In a separate cup, dissolve chocolate in hot coffee. Stir until combined. Pour espresso sauce over other ingredients. Serve.

NOTE: Most commercial ice creams are synthetic concoctions that contain little milk and no eggs. When buying ice cream, choose those brands which list ingredients on the package and which contain no artificial colors, flavors and texturizers. An alternative is to make your own ice cream or ice milk at home, either with an ice-cream machine or the old-fashioned way by hand. Most basic cookbooks give instructions. Real ice cream can provide good nutrition, especially protein, but should not be relied on exclusively as a milk source because of its high sugar content.

FISH BISQUE

MAKES: 4 bowls
PROTEIN: 18 grams per bowl

> ¼ cup onion, diced
> 3 tablespoons butter
> 2 cups canned salmon, deboned and flaked
> 3 cups Cream Sauce (see page 174)
> 3 tablespoons sherry
> Milk, heated
> Paprika and chives

In a large saucepan, sauté onions in butter until they are transparent. Add the salmon and cream sauce. Stirring constantly, bring to boiling point, but do not boil.

Remove from heat and add sherry. Add milk to desired thinness. Garnish with paprika and chives. Serve hot.

*To vary, substitute for salmon an equal amount of tuna, diced shrimp, crab meat, lobster or minced clams.

NEW ENGLAND CLAM CHOWDER

MAKES: 4 bowls
PROTEIN: 23 grams per bowl

> *3-inch cube salt pork or 3 strips bacon*
> *½ cup onion, diced*
> *2 cups potatoes, diced*
> *2 tablespoons whole-wheat flour*
> *½ teaspoon salt*
> *Pepper*
> *3 bay leaves*
> *Clam juice*
> *3 cups fresh or canned clams, coarsely chopped*
> *2 cups milk, heated*
> *Butter*

Cook salt pork or bacon in a large saucepan until fat is released, then remove. Stir onions into drippings and cook until just soft.

Place potatoes in a bowl and sprinkle with the flour, salt, and pepper. Add to onions along with bay leaves and juice from the clams. If needed, add enough hot water to cover potatoes and simmer until potatoes are tender, but not mushy.

Add clams, bring to a boil, and cook 2 more minutes. Do not overcook or clams will be leathery.

Stir in heated milk and a few chunks of butter. Remove from heat and let stand until butter melts. Remove bay leaves before serving. The traditional accompaniment is Oysterettes or saltine crackers.

PUMPKIN PIE

MAKES: 1 8-slice pie
PROTEIN: 8 grams per slice

Whole-Wheat Piecrust

> *1 cup whole-wheat flour*
> *¼ cup wheat germ*
> *1 teaspoon salt*
> *⅓ cup corn oil*
> *3 tablespoons milk*

In a bowl, combine flour, wheat germ and salt. Add oil and milk to dry ingredients and mix lightly with a fork until mixture is moistened, but not sticky.

Press dough evenly into an oiled 8- or 9-inch pie plate, making as high a rim as possible.

For pumpkin pie, do not pre-bake. If being used for a pie that requires a pre-baked shell, crust should bake for 8 minutes at 475°.

Filling

> *6 eggs*
> *1 16-ounce can unsweetened pumpkin (not pie mix)*
> *½ cup honey*
> *½ teaspoon salt*
> *2 teaspoons cinnamon*
> *1 teaspoon ginger*
> *½ teaspoon cloves*
> *1 cup evaporated milk*

In a large bowl, beat eggs until fluffy. Add pumpkin and mix thoroughly, then add all other ingredients. Stir until mixture is even-colored, with no streaks.

Pour into an unbaked shell and bake for 15 minutes at 425°, then reduce heat to 350° and bake another 45 minutes, or until done. A knife inserted into center will come out clean when done. Cool before serving. Top with whipped cream.

RICE PUDDING

MAKES: 5 cups
PROTEIN: 10 grams per cup

> 2 cups cooked brown rice
> 2½ cups milk
> ½ cup powdered milk
> ⅓ cup honey
> 3 tablespoons butter
> 2 teaspoons vanilla
> 4 eggs, beaten
> 1 cup raisins
> 1 teaspoon cinnamon
> ½ teaspoon salt

Preheat oven to 350°. Butter a quart-and-a-half baking dish or casserole.

Combine all ingredients in a large bowl. Pour into baking dish and bake about 40 minutes, or until set. Knife inserted into center will come out clean when done.

Custard will rise to top. If you prefer to have it mixed through pudding, stir two or three times while pudding is baking.

Serve warm or chilled.

SPINACH SOUFFLÉ

MAKES: 4 servings
PROTEIN: 16 grams per serving

> *1 cup Cream Sauce (see page 174)*
> *4 egg yolks*
> *1 cup Cheddar cheese, coarsely grated*
> *3 tablespoons parsley*
> *3 tablespoons onion, minced*
> *6 egg whites, beaten stiff*
> *3 cups dry raw spinach, chopped fine*

Preheat oven to 350°.

Heat cream sauce, then pour into a large bowl. Add egg yolks, cheese, parsley and onion and mix thoroughly. Fold in egg whites gently until no streaks of egg or cheese are left. Sprinkle spinach, a handful at a time, into mixture and combine gently.

Pour mixture into a buttered deep baking dish or casserole. A springform pan can be used successfully. Bake 40 minutes or until set.

Serve at once, as the soufflé falls rapidly after leaving oven.

VICHYSSOISE

MAKES: 4 bowls
PROTEIN: 8 grams per bowl

> *4 leeks or onions, minced (about 1½ cups)*
> *3 tablespoons butter*
> *1½ cups potatoes, thinly sliced*
> *1½ cups chicken broth*
> *½ cup powdered milk*
> *1 cup milk*
> *½ cup sour cream*
> *Chives, chopped*

In a saucepan, sauté leeks or onions in butter until soft. Add potatoes and chicken broth, cover and simmer for 20 minutes, or until potatoes are very soft.

Pour potato mixture into blender with powdered milk and blend 10 seconds on medium speed.

Return to saucepan and add milk and sour cream. Stir thoroughly, then place in refrigerator to chill.

Serve garnished with chives.

WELSH RAREBIT

MAKES: 6 servings
PROTEIN: 20 grams per serving

> *1 tablespoon butter*
> *1 pound sharp Cheddar cheese, grated*
> *1 cup beer*
> *1 teaspoon dry mustard*
> *Water*
> *Pepper to taste*
> *2 egg yolks*

In a saucepan or chafing dish, melt butter and cheese. Add beer when cheese is partially melted, stirring until well mixed.

Mix mustard with a small amount of water to form a soft paste. Add to cheese mixture along with pepper.

When mixture is slightly thickened, remove from heat and stir in egg yolks. Serve hot on whole-wheat toast or English muffins.

II.
Meat, Poultry and Seafood

BAKED COD FILLET

MAKES: 4 servings
PROTEIN: 36 grams per serving

> 4 six-ounce fillets of fresh codfish
> ¾ cup wheat germ
> Mayonnaise

Preheat oven to 400°. Grease a large glass baking dish.

Spread both sides of each fillet generously with mayonnaise and coat with wheat germ. Bake for 15 minutes or until the cod starts to separate into large chunks when touched with a fork.

BEEF FONDUE

MAKES: 4 servings
PROTEIN: 30 grams per serving

> 1½ pounds beef sirloin, ¾-inch cubes
> 1 cup unsalted butter or corn oil

Melt butter in a fondue pot, chafing dish or saucepan over flame adequate to keep cooking heat constant. Spear one or two cubes of beef on long, sharp-tined forks and swirl in butter when it starts to turn brown. The meat cooks rapidly, so be careful not to leave it in too long or it will be quite tough. Dip the meat in sauces arranged on each plate.

Sauces

Cream sauce (see page 174) with 2 teaspoons curry powder per cup

Ketchup with 1 teaspoon Worcestershire sauce and 2 teaspoons minced onion per cup

Prepared mustard with 3 teaspoons chopped parsley and 1 teaspoon sage per cup

Mayonnaise with 2 teaspoons anchovy paste and 1 teaspoon garlic powder per cup

Welsh rarebit (see page 162)

BERMUDA SCALLOPS

MAKES: 4 servings
PROTEIN: 28 grams per serving

> 1¼ pounds bay scallops
> 3 tablespoons corn oil
> 3 tablespoons lemon juice
> ½ teaspoon ground cloves
> ¼ cup onion, minced
> ¼ cup fresh parsley, chopped
> 3 tablespoons butter

Marinate the scallops for one hour in a large skillet with oil, lemon juice and cloves, turning two or three times.

Add the onions, parsley and butter and cook over medium heat for 15 minutes or until the scallops begin to release their juices. Serve immediately with sauce.

Sauce

> 1 cup cooled Cream Sauce (see page 174)
> 2 egg yolks, beaten
> ⅛ teaspoon dry mustard
> 1 teaspoon vinegar
> 2 tablespoons fresh parsley, chopped

In a saucepan over low heat add egg yolks, mustard and vinegar to cream sauce. Mix thoroughly and remove from heat just before the mixture is about to boil. Add the parsley and pour over scallops.

BOUILLABAISSE

MAKES: 10 bowls
PROTEIN: 59 grams per serving

1 pound each (cleaned and cut into 2-inch pieces): flounder, perch, haddock, cod, shrimp, or any other fish available
1 pound hard-shell clams
2 dozen live mussels, washed
1½ cups onions, minced
1 teaspoon garlic powder
1 cup tomato purée
1 cup whole tomatoes, peeled and chopped
2 bay leaves
1 teaspoon thyme
1 three-inch strip of orange rind
6 whole cloves
½ cup olive oil
¼ teaspoon saffron (optional)
2 quarts water

In a large soup pot, place all the ingredients except the clams, shrimp, mussels and water. Swirl the pot so that the fish is well covered with liquid. Add water and bring to a brisk, rolling boil over high heat. Boil for 8 minutes. Add the clams, shrimp and mussels and boil another 8 minutes, or until mussels open.

Serve the fish on a separate platter. The broth is served over thick slices of bread in soup bowls.

CRÊPES LAKE FOREST

MAKES: 4 filled crêpes
PROTEIN: 9 grams per piece

Batter

> *1 egg*
> *½ cup milk*
> *⅛ teaspoon salt*
> *1 teaspoon corn oil*
> *⅓ cup whole-wheat flour*

Combine all the ingredients in a bowl. Drop by the tablespoon onto an oiled, hot skillet or crêpe pan. Do not overcrowd because mixture spreads widely. After one minute, turn and cook the other side until golden. Stack crêpes until ready for filling.

Filling

> *2 tablespoons butter*
> *2 tablespoons whole-wheat flour*
> *½ cup chicken broth*
> *½ cup milk*
> *2 tablespoons dry white wine*
> *½ cup cooked mushrooms*
> *½ cup Swiss cheese, grated*
> *½ cup cooked chicken*
> *¼ cup fresh parsley, chopped*

Melt the butter in a medium-sized saucepan. Add flour and stir for one minute. Then add broth, milk and wine. Blend until smooth.

In a separate bowl, combine the remaining ingredients and stir into sauce.

To assemble crêpes, place ⅓ cup of filling into center of each crêpe. Roll into a tube shape and turn ends under. Serve hot.

ITALIAN SWEET SAUSAGE IN PASTRY

MAKES: 12 sausages
PROTEIN: 9 grams each

12 Italian sweet sausages, 4-inch links, thoroughly cooked

Whole-Wheat Pastry Crust

> *2 cups whole-wheat flour*
> *½ cup soy flour*
> *⅓ cup cream cheese*
> *⅓ cup butter*
> *3 eggs, beaten*
> *½ teaspoon salt*
> *Cold water*

Place all the wheat and soy flour in a bowl. Using a table fork or fingertips, cut in the cheese and butter until mixture resembles small beads. Stir in the eggs and salt until dough forms a ball and leaves the sides of bowl clean. Depending on flour used, a few tablespoons of water may be needed to achieve correct degree of firmness and smoothness.

Chill pastry for 30 minutes, then preheat oven to 375°. Roll out dough on a floured surface to ½-inch thickness. Cut into ob- longs large enough to cover sausage, overlapping the sides and tucking ends under.

With the seam edge down, place on an oiled baking sheet and bake for 25 minutes or until pastry is lightly browned.

Serve hot with Mustard Sauce (page 176).

NOTE: The best place to buy Italian sausage is at a store that makes its own fresh every day and does not use any additives to preserve or color the meat. My mother and aunts still prefer to make their own sausage at home. Italian specialty stores often make their own. Supermarkets generally do not, but ask the manager what their brands contain, as they often lack labels.

LASAGNA

MAKES: 8 servings
PROTEIN: 56 grams per serving

Noodles

1½ pound high-protein lasagna noodles (Buitoni brand)
2 tablespoons olive oil

Italian Tomato Sauce

¼ cup olive oil
1 cup onions, chopped
1 teaspoon garlic powder
2 six-ounce cans tomato paste
6 cups tomato purée
3 tablespoons sweet basil
3 tablespoons oregano
Pepper
2 cups water

Filling

> 1 pound mozzarella cheese, sliced
> 2 pounds ricotta cheese
> ¼ pound Parmesan cheese, grated
> 2 pounds ground beef, cooked and drained

Cook noodles according to package directions adding 2 tablespoons of oil to prevent sticking.

In a large saucepan sauté the onions in olive oil until soft. Add garlic powder and tomato paste and stir continually until the oil is blended into the paste. Add the remaining sauce ingredients and bring to a boil. Reduce heat and simmer 30 minutes. Preheat oven to 375°.

To assemble lasagna, spoon 1 cup of sauce into the bottom of a large baking pan, at least 2 inches deep. Place lasagna noodles side by side, slightly overlapping them, until the bottom of pan is covered. Coat noodles with more sauce. Spread half the ground beef on the noodles, then cover with sauce. Spread half the ricotta cheese next, then cover with sauce. Make another layer of noodles, then all the mozzarella and Parmesan, followed by sauce, meat, sauce, ricotta, sauce, finishing with noodles and sauce. Bake 45 minutes. Serve hot.

LIVER PÂTÉ ANDERSON

MAKES: 2 cups
PROTEIN: 100 grams per cup

> *1 pound chicken livers*
> *2 medium onions*
> *2 tablespoons butter*
> *2 hard-boiled eggs, mashed*
> *2 tablespoons water*
> *Salt and pepper*

Broil the livers 5 minutes on each side or until middles are no longer pink.

Sauté the onions in butter, then place in a bowl, reserving drippings in onion pan. Add the liver and eggs and grind or mash until finely mixed.

Add water to onion drippings, then add to liver mixture a spoonful at a time until it reaches the consistency of spreadable paste. Season to taste. Serve with crackers or as sandwich filling.

REUBEN SANDWICH

MAKES: 1 sandwich
PROTEIN: 30 grams per sandwich

> *2 slices rye bread, toasted and buttered*
> *2 ounces corned beef, thinly sliced*
> *2 ounces Swiss cheese*
> *½ cup sauerkraut*
> *Salt and pepper*

Place the corned beef and cheese on one slice of toast. Place under the broiler or in a toaster oven until cheese begins to melt. Remove from heat, add sauerkraut and top with other slice of toast. Serve hot.

SHRIMP SCAMPI

MAKES: 4 servings
PROTEIN: 30 grams per serving

> 1½ pounds small shrimp, cleaned
> ¾ cup melted butter
> Garlic powder
> Paprika
> Salt and pepper

Butter a flat baking sheet or shallow glass baking pan. Arrange shrimp in a single layer and pour melted butter over them. Sprinkle with garlic powder, paprika, salt and pepper.

Place under the broiler and cook until shrimps turn pink, basting occasionally with the seasoned butter.

Serve hot.

SPAGHETTI AND MEATBALLS

MAKES: 4 servings
PROTEIN: 40 grams per serving

> 1 pound high-protein or whole-wheat spaghetti (Buitoni)
> 2 tablespoons olive oil
> 6 cups Italian Tomato Sauce (see page 168)

Meatballs

> *1 pound ground beef*
> *1 cup bread crumbs*
> *2 eggs*
> *¼ cup fresh parsley, chopped*
> *¼ cup Parmesan cheese*

Cook spaghetti according to the package instructions, adding oil to keep pasta from sticking. Prepare the sauce.

Combine all meatball ingredients in a bowl and mix thoroughly. Shape into balls about 2 inches across.

In a large skillet, heat olive oil and fry meatballs until well browned on all sides.

Drain on paper towels, then place into a large saucepan with the tomato sauce and simmer for 30 minutes.

Place the cooked spaghetti on a large platter or individual dishes, put meatballs on the side and cover both with tomato sauce. Serve hot with grated Parmesan cheese.

TUNA ROMA

MAKES: 4 servings
PROTEIN: 25 grams per serving

1 cup egg noodles, cooked
2 cups canned tuna, drained
⅓ cup dry white wine
2 cups fresh green peas, cooked
(frozen may be substituted
in winter)

½ cup fresh parsley, chopped
¾ cup Italian Tomato Sauce
(see page 168)
Salt and pepper

Place all the ingredients in a saucepan, heat and serve.

TURKEY POT PIE

MAKES: 6 servings
PROTEIN: 21 grams per serving

1½ cups chicken broth	*4 hard-boiled eggs, sliced*
½ cup sweet corn	*½ cup fresh parsley, chopped*
½ cup peas	*2 cups Cream Sauce*
½ cup carrots, diced	*(see page 174)*
1 cup potatoes, diced	*1 Whole-Wheat Pastry Crust*
1 cup onions, diced	*(see page 167)*
2 cups turkey, cooked and diced	

In a saucepan simmer corn, peas, carrots, potatoes and onions in broth for 15 minutes.

Add turkey, eggs, parsley and cream sauce and heat over medium heat for 5 minutes.

Preheat oven to 400°. Butter a deep baking dish or casserole.

Spoon mixture into the baking dish and place pastry shell crust, cut to fit and rolled to ½ inch thick, over top. Make several slashes in pastry to allow steam to escape during baking.

Bake for 30 minutes or until pastry is browned. Serve with crust on bottom and turkey mixture spooned over top.

III.
Sauces and Dressings

CREAM SAUCE

MAKES: 2 cups
PROTEIN: 9 grams per cup

> *4 tablespoons butter*
> *4 tablespoons whole-wheat flour*
> *2 cups milk*
> *Salt and pepper*

Melt the butter in a saucepan. Sprinkle in flour and stir quickly to form a heavy paste. Add milk ¼ cup at a time, stirring so that sauce becomes smooth. Continue to stir gently as sauce thickens to desired consistency. Salt and pepper to taste.

Cream sauce is the basis for many soups and may be used plain with vegetables, poultry and some seafood, or in pot pies.

There are numerous variations of cream sauce which can be found in basic cookbooks. One of the most valuable of these variations is:

CHEESE SAUCE

MAKES: 3 cups
PROTEIN: 15 grams per cup

> *2 cups cream sauce*
> *1½ cups sharp, aged cheese, grated*
> *Paprika*

Add cheese to sauce after milk, stirring until blended. Garnish with paprika.

CHOCOLATE SAUCE

MAKES: 2 cups
PROTEIN: 11 grams per cup

>*4 ounces unsweetened chocolate squares*
>*2 tablespoons butter*
>*⅔ cup evaporated milk*
>*1 cup honey*
>*¼ cup water*
>*2 eggs, beaten until fluffy*
>*2 teaspoons vanilla or rum*

In a fondue pot or saucepan, place the chocolate squares, butter and milk, stirring over medium heat until chocolate and butter melt.

In a separate pan heat the honey and water until thinned. Add three tablespoons of honey mixture to eggs, then pour the remaining honey and eggs into chocolate mixture. Mix thoroughly. Add vanilla or rum just before serving. The sauce should be satiny and glossy.

If used as a dessert fondue, sauce may need to be thinned occasionally with a small amount of milk in order to maintain proper dipping consistency.

MUSTARD SAUCE

MAKES: 1 cup
PROTEIN: 6 grams per cup

> ¾ cup sour cream
> ¼ cup prepared mustard
> 2 tablespoons vinegar
> 2 tablespoons corn oil
> Salt and pepper

Mix all the ingredients in a small bowl.
Serve over salad greens or as a dip for hors d'oeuvres.

OIL AND VINEGAR DRESSING

MAKES: 1 cup
PROTEIN: none

> ½ cup olive oil
> 3 tablespoons wine vinegar
> Salt and pepper

Stir thoroughly in a cup or shake in a covered jar until oil
and vinegar mix. Dressing should be made fresh for each salad.
To vary, add any one of these combinations:

2 tablespoons tarragon and 1 hard-boiled egg
2 tablespoons basil and 1 teaspoon oregano
1 tablespoon capers and 1 teaspoon anchovy paste
2 tablespoons rosemary and 2 tablespoons orange juice concentrate
1 teaspoon garlic powder and 2 teaspoons minced onion
2 teaspoons celery seeds and 2 teaspoons dill

ORANGE SAUCE

MAKES: 1½ cups
PROTEIN: none

>   ¾ cup honey
>   4 tablespoons orange-juice concentrate
>   Peel of one orange, finely grated
>   ½ cup canned apricots, puréed

Heat all the ingredients in a small saucepan over medium heat until honey is thinned. Stir occasionally. Serve warm. May also be used as a glaze for poultry.

ROQUEFORT DRESSING

MAKES: 1 cup
PROTEIN: 12 grams per cup

>   ½ cup sour cream
>   ¼ cup Roquefort or blue cheese
>   ¼ cup plain yoghurt
>   3 tablespoons lemon juice
>   Pepper

Combine all ingredients in a small bowl. Serve over salad greens or as a dip for raw vegetables.

YOGHURT DRESSING

MAKES: 1 cup
PROTEIN: 8 grams per cup

> ¾ cup plain yoghurt
> 3 tablespoons tomato paste
> ¼ cup chopped parsley
> 1 tablespoon lemon juice
> Pepper

Combine all the ingredients in a small bowl. Serve over salad greens or as a dip for raw vegetables.

IV.
Breads and Grains

BRAN MUFFINS

MAKES: 12 muffins
PROTEIN: 3.5 grams per muffin

> 2 cups whole-wheat flour
> 1 cup wheat bran or 100% bran flakes
> 1½ teaspoons baking soda
> ½ teaspoon salt
> 1½ cups plain yoghurt
> 2 eggs, beaten
> ¼ cup molasses

Preheat oven to 375°. Oil or butter muffin pans.

Combine flour, bran, soda and salt in a bowl. Mix thoroughly. Add the remaining ingredients and beat until mixed well.

Fill muffin cups about ⅔ full. Bake for 30 minutes or until a knife inserted comes out clean.

To vary, add up to ½ cup raisins or chopped dates to batter.

BLUEBERRY MUFFINS

Follow recipe for Bran Muffins.

Substitute 1 cup of blueberries for bran flakes and ½ cup of honey for molasses.

CHEESE POPCORN

MAKES: 4 cups
PROTEIN: 4 grams per cup

> ½ cup popcorn kernels
> Corn oil
> ¼ cup butter, melted
> ¼ cup Parmesan cheese
> Salt

In a large saucepan, place oil to depth of ¼ inch and add 3 or 4 kernels of popcorn. Place over medium high heat. When test kernels pop, add the rest of the corn, shaking occasionally as it pops.

Turn out popped corn into a large bowl. In a saucepan, melt butter and pour it over corn. Add Parmesan and salt to taste. Toss well so that cheese and salt are evenly distributed. Serve hot.

FRENCH STRAWBERRY PANCAKES

MAKES: 12 filled pancakes
PROTEIN: 2.5 grams per pancake

> *3 cups fresh strawberries*
> *½ cup honey*

Follow recipe for Cheese Blintz batter (see page 140) and place on a warm serving platter.

Put strawberries in a saucepan.

Add the honey and warm over low heat.

Fill pancakes and serve hot with Orange Sauce (see page 177).

HIGH-PROTEIN BROWNIES

MAKES: 12 brownies
PROTEIN: 8 grams per brownie

> *½ cup butter*
> *1 cup honey*
> *1 tablespoon vanilla*
> *½ cup evaporated milk*
> *½ cup powdered milk*
> *⅓ cup cocoa*
> *1¼ cups wheat germ*
> *½ teaspoon baking powder*
> *½ teaspoon salt*
> *1½ cups walnut pieces*

Preheat oven to 325°. Oil baking pan (8 by 8 inches or 8 by 11 inches).

Melt butter in a saucepan over medium-low heat. Remove from heat and add honey. Stir thoroughly, then add vanilla.

In a separate cup combine powdered and evaporated milk and stir until lumps disappear. Add milk to honey mixture, then stir in cocoa, mixing thoroughly. Add remaining ingredients and pour into a baking pan.

Bake for 25 minutes or until a knife inserted comes out clean. Cool in pan and cut into pieces. Serve with cream cheese, ice cream or plain with milk for a snack.

If you prefer a more fudgey brownie, omit the baking powder.

HIGH-PROTEIN GRANOLA

MAKES: 20 cups
PROTEIN: 15 grams per cup

> *7 cups rolled oats*
> *2 cups peanuts, salted*
> *2 cups pecans or almonds, chopped*
> *1 cup sunflower seeds*
> *1½ cups powdered milk*
> *1 cup shredded coconut, unsweetened*
> *1 cup wheat germ*
> *1⅔ cups peanut butter, natural*
> *¾ cup corn oil*
> *1 cup honey*
> *2 tablespoons vanilla*
> *½ cup water*

Preheat oven to 375°. Oil a very large roasting pan and mix all dry ingredients in it.

In a saucepan over medium heat, mix peanut butter, oil, honey, vanilla and water.

Pour liquid mixture over dry ingredients and mix thoroughly until everything is just moistened. A few extra sprinkles of water may be needed if oats are very dry.

Bake until oats are golden brown, stirring every 5 minutes so that sides and bottom don't stick and burn. When done, open oven door and let cool in pan. Mixture forms small chunks as it dries. Store in a covered container.

Serve plain as a snack, with yoghurt or milk and fresh fruit for breakfast or dessert, or crumbled over ice cream or pudding as a topping.

HIGH-PROTEIN PANCAKES

MAKES: 9 5-inch pancakes
PROTEIN: 4 grams per pancake

> ¾ cup whole-wheat flour
> ¼ cup soy flour
> ½ cup powdered milk
> 1 teaspoon baking powder
> ½ teaspoon salt
> ¼ cup shredded coconut, unsweetened
> 1 cup milk
> 2 eggs
> ¼ cup corn oil

In a bowl, combine all dry ingredients. Add milk, eggs and oil. Stir thoroughly until lumps disappear. A bit of extra milk or water may be added if batter is too thick, or if it thickens in the bowl while some pancakes are being cooked. It should be the consistency of a thick creamed soup.

Pour just enough oil in a large skillet to coat surface lightly. For each pancake, pour 3 tablespoons of batter slowly onto the skillet over medium-high heat. Turn when bubbles rise to surface in center and bottom is browned.

Stack pancakes and keep warm in oven at 200° until ready to serve. Serve with butter and maple syrup or honey.

PEANUT BUTTER COOKIES

MAKES: 2 dozen 3-inch cookies
PROTEIN: 2 grams per cookie

> *1½ cups whole-wheat flour*
> *½ cup powdered milk*
> *½ teaspoon baking soda*
> *1 teaspoon baking powder*
> *½ teaspoon salt*
> *1 cup natural peanut butter*
> *½ cup honey*
> *2 eggs, beaten*
> *¼ cup butter, melted*
> *1 teaspoon vanilla*

Preheat oven to 375°. Oil a baking sheet.

Combine all dry ingredients in a bowl. Add remaining ingredients and mix thoroughly. Dough will be stiff.

For each cookie, drop two tablespoons of dough on a baking sheet. With wet fork tines, press top of cookie once to flatten, then again at right angles to make pattern of squares on top. Leave room between cookies for them to swell a bit as they bake.

Bake for 15 minutes or until just lightly browned. Cookies should not be hardened. Remove from oven and cool on the baking sheet. Store in closed container so that cookies stay moist.

SUSAN'S BUTTERMILK BISCUITS

MAKES: 18 2-inch biscuits
PROTEIN: 3 grams per biscuit

> 2 cups whole-wheat flour
> ¼ cup wheat germ
> 2 teaspoons baking powder
> ½ teaspoon baking soda
> ½ teaspoon salt
> 5 tablespoons butter, hard, in small pieces
> 1¼ cup buttermilk

Preheat oven to 400°.

In a bowl, combine dry ingredients. Add butter and work in with fork until mixture is crumbly. Mix in buttermilk. Dough will be soft, but hold together.

Turn out on a floured surface and pat 1 inch thick. Cut with a biscuit cutter and place on an ungreased baking sheet.

Bake 10 to 15 minutes or until tops begin to brown. Serve hot.

VERMONT BROWN BREAD

MAKES: 2 large 9-by-5-inch loaves
PROTEIN: 115 grams per loaf

3¾ cups very warm water
½ cup plus 1 tablespoon honey
2 tablespoons dry yeast
(2 packages)
1 egg, beaten until foamy
⅓ cup corn oil
2 teaspoons salt

2 cups rolled oats
1 cup cracked wheat (bulgur)
1 cup wheat germ
1 cup soy flour
1 cup rye flour
2 cups powdered milk
7–8 cups whole-wheat flour

Into ½ cup of the water, stir 1 tablespoon of the honey, then the yeast. Let settle, then stir again. Allow to sit in a warm place for 10 minutes until yeast is completely dissolved. Mixture should form bubbles as yeast begins to "work." If it does not, yeast is not active, so begin again with fresh ingredients.

In a large soup pot, mix remaining water, honey, egg, oil and salt, stirring after each addition. Add yeast mixture, then all dry ingredients, except 3 cups whole wheat flour. Mix thoroughly until dough is quite sticky, and getting hard to stir.

Use 1 cup of flour to cover a large working surface. Turn dough out on it and sprinkle more flour over dough surface. Let rest 10 minutes before beginning to knead it.

Knead the dough for 10 minutes, adding one or more cups of flour, a bit at a time, to keep the dough covered with a thin layer of unabsorbed flour. This helps keep dough from sticking to hands and work surface. If dough does begin to stick, just scrape the bits up, add them back to large dough mass and continue to knead.

Toward the end of the 10 minutes, you will notice a greater resistance to your handling. Stop adding flour and knead until all the excess flour on the dough mass is absorbed.

Oil a pot at least twice as large as the dough mass. Place the dough in, then turn it over so that its top is oiled. This keeps dough from forming a crust as it rises.

Cover with a wet cloth and place in a warm spot (inside an unlighted oven is usually good) for 2 to 3 hours until doubled in bulk.

Punch dough down inside pot, forcing out trapped air bubbles. Turn out on a lightly floured work surface and divide dough in two. Flatten each piece and pat into rectangular shape.

Grease two loaf pans. Place dough loaves into pans. Cover with a damp cloth and return to warm place to rise for 1 hour.

Preheat oven to 400°. Bake bread for 15 minutes, then reduce heat to 325° and bake at least 45 more minutes. Do not open oven door to check bread until it has been baking for at least 30 minutes. When done, bread will sound hollow when tapped.

Turn out and cool upside down on a rack. Store in aluminum foil or plastic bags, but do not wrap until bread is thoroughly cool. This bread provides three times the protein of store-bought white bread.

WHOLE-WHEAT BUNS

MAKES: 8 hamburger-size buns
PROTEIN: 7 grams per bun

> *1 cup very warm water*
> *1 tablespoon dry yeast (1 package)*
> *1 tablespoon honey*
> *3 cups whole-wheat flour*
> *½ cup powdered milk*
> *1 teaspoon salt*
> *¼ cup corn oil*
> *1 egg, beaten*
> *¼ cup melted butter*
> *Sesame seeds*

In a cup, mix honey and water. Sprinkle in yeast. Combine and let stand 5 to 10 minutes until foamy. If bubbles do not appear, yeast is not active and you must begin again with fresh ingredients.

Place dry ingredients in a bowl and stir in yeast mixture. Add oil and egg. Mix thoroughly.

Turn out on a floured surface and knead for five minutes. Pat to 1 inch thick and cut with a 3-inch bun cutter. Brush melted butter on tops and sprinkle with sesame seeds. Place on oiled baking sheet. Let rise for approximately two hours or until almost doubled in bulk.

Preheat oven to 350°. Bake for 15 to 20 minutes or until lightly browned.

Cool on a rack. Slice in half and serve with hamburgers or sandwich filling.

V.
Fruits

AMBROSIA

MAKES: 4 cups
PROTEIN: 2 grams per cup

⅔ cup pineapple chunks
⅔ cup grapefruit sections
⅔ cup bananas, sliced
⅔ cup apples, chopped
⅔ cup peaches, cut up

⅔ cup dates, pitted
½ cup shredded coconut,
   unsweetened
⅔ cup orange juice

Combine all the fruit in a serving dish. Spoon juice over. Serve chilled.

APRICOTS IN HONEY CREAM

MAKES: 4 servings
PROTEIN: 5.5 grams per serving

> 2 cups apricots, fresh or canned in fruit juice
> ¾ cup heavy cream
> ½ cup milk
> ½ cup powdered milk
> 3 tablespoons honey

Cut apricots in pieces and place in a serving dish. In a separate cup, dissolve powdered milk in cream and whole milk. Stir in honey. Pour cream mixture over apricots and serve chilled.

AVOCADO-GRAPEFRUIT SALAD

MAKES: 4 servings
PROTEIN: 3 grams per serving

> 2 grapefruits, sectioned
> 2 avocados, cut in slivers
> Mayonnaise
> Walnuts, chopped
> Lettuce leaves

Arrange grapefruit and avocado sections on a bed of lettuce. Top with a dollop of mayonnaise and sprinkle with walnuts. Serve chilled.

BAKED APPLE, BONNE FEMME

MAKES: 4 servings
PROTEIN: 2 to 4 grams per serving, depending on bread used

4 tart apples, cored and peeled ⅓ way down sides
4 slices whole-grain bread, buttered and sprinkled with cinnamon
4 tablespoons butter
4 teaspoons cinnamon
Honey

Preheat oven to 375°. Butter a shallow baking pan.

Arrange bread slices in pan. Place 1 apple on each slice of bread. Push 1 tablespoon butter into bottom of each apple center. Spoon in 1 teaspoon cinnamon. Fill the remainder of each apple center with honey.

Bake for 30 minutes or until tender, but not mushy.

Serve warm or chilled with milk or cream.

BANANAS BALTIMORE

MAKES: 4 cups
PROTEIN: 6 grams per cup

3 bananas, sliced
1 teaspoon garam masala *
¼ teaspoon chili powder
Pinch of dried red chili peppers
¼ teaspoon salt
3 cups plain yoghurt
Anise seeds

* This spice may be obtained in Indian specialty stores.

Blend all seasonings (except anise seeds) with yoghurt in a bowl. Add bananas and stir. Garnish with anise seeds.

Chill tightly covered for ½ hour.

BROILED PEACH AMANDINE

MAKES: 4 servings
PROTEIN: 1 gram per serving

8 peach halves, peeled
8 tablespoons honey
8 teaspoons butter
4 teaspoons rum
Almond slivers, toasted

Place peach halves on a buttered baking dish. Distribute honey, butter and rum evenly among them.

Broil 3 inches from heat until butter melts and peaches are warmed. Serve immediately, garnished with almonds.

CITRUS PUNCH

MAKES: 1 quart
PROTEIN: none

> *1 cup light tea*
> *Juice of 1 lemon*
> *2 cups pineapple juice*
> *½ cup orange juice*
> *½ cup grapefruit juice*
> *Fresh strawberries, halved*
> *Shaved ice*

Stir all the liquids together. Add a few strawberry halves to each glass and serve over ice.

CRANBERRY-ORANGE RELISH

MAKES: 2 cups
PROTEIN: none

> *1½ cups fresh cranberries, chopped*
> *½ cup orange juice concentrate*
> *½ cup yellow raisins*
> *Peel of two oranges, slivered*
> *Honey to taste (about ½ cup)*

Combine all ingredients in a bowl. Place in glass jars and store, covered, in the refrigerator for at least two days before serving.

FRESH FRUIT TART

MAKES: 6 servings
PROTEIN: 13 grams per serving

Crust

> *1 recipe Whole-Wheat Pastry Crust (see page 167)*
> *½ cup shredded coconut, unsweetened*

Add coconut to whole-wheat pastry, then refrigerate for 30 minutes.

Preheat oven to 400°. Butter an 8-inch pie tin.

Roll out the dough on a lightly floured surface. Lift into the tin and finish edge by crimping or rolling it over slightly. Prick surface of crust with fork. Bake for 12 minutes or until crust is lightly browned. Remove from the oven and let cool to room temperature. Reset oven to 325°.

Filling

> *3 cups fresh fruit (mixed or one variety)*
> *½ cup honey*
> *¼ cup apple juice, hot*
> *1 tablespoon gelatin (1 package)*

Cut fruit up into small pieces, peeled or unpeeled. Add honey and mix until fruit pieces are coated. Place fruit mixture into baked crust.

In a separate cup, dissolve gelatin in apple juice. Brush mixture over top of fruit in tart. This seals fruit and helps prevent discoloration if tart is not served at once.

Meringue

> 4 egg whites
> ½ teaspoon cream of tartar
> ⅓ cup honey

In a bowl, beat egg whites with an electric mixer until very stiff. Add cream of tartar, then the honey 1 tablespoon at a time, until egg whites are glossy and stand in peaks. Oil brown paper and use it to line bottom of a baking sheet. Drop some egg white mixture onto paper with a large serving spoon, lifting up the spoon tip in center of each puff to make a peak. Immediately place puffs in the oven and bake for 20 minutes or until meringues are dry. They need not become brown in order to be done. Turn off oven and allow meringues to cool on baking sheet with oven door open.

Use to decorate top of tart, either by arranging around the outside edge or by covering the entire top.

FRUIT CURRY

MAKES: 4 servings
PROTEIN: 1 gram per serving

> 2 bananas, sliced
> 1 cup pineapple chunks
> 1 cup cantaloupe, in small pieces
> Juice of 1 lemon
> ½ cup pineapple juice
> 1 teaspoon curry powder

In a serving bowl, slice bananas and squeeze lemon juice over them to prevent discoloration. Add the rest of the fruit and combine.

In a cup, stir curry powder into pineapple juice, then pour over fruit in bowl. Serve chilled.

FRUIT FONDUE

MAKES: 6 servings
PROTEIN: 5 grams per serving

> *3 fresh pears, sliced*
> *3 fresh peaches, sliced*
> *2 cups sweet cherries, pitted*
> *1 recipe Chocolate Sauce (see page 175)*

Arrange the fruit on individual dessert plates. Heat the sauce in a fondue pot or chafing dish. Using long-handled, sharp-tined forks, spear fruit, one piece at a time, and swirl in sauce until covered. Allow the sauce to harden a bit on the fruit before eating.

GRAPE DELIGHT

MAKES: 4 servings
PROTEIN: 7 grams per serving

> *2 cups seedless green grapes, chopped*
> *1 cup pistachios or almonds, chopped*
> *¾ cup plain yoghurt*
> *¼ cup honey*
> *Candied ginger*

Combine grapes and nuts in a serving dish. Toss with yoghurt and honey. Sprinkle ginger over the top and serve.

PEACH UPSIDE-DOWN CAKE

MAKES: 8 pieces
PROTEIN: 4 grams per piece

*2½ cups fresh or canned
    peaches, peeled and sliced*
½ cup honey
1 lemon
1 teaspoon cinnamon
1½ cups whole-wheat flour
½ cup wheat germ

2 teaspoons baking powder
½ teaspoon salt
2 eggs
2 egg yolks
¼ cup butter
⅓ cup evaporated milk
Sour cream or whipped cream

Preheat oven to 425°. Butter a deep, straight-sided casserole that holds at least 2 quarts.

Place peaches in the bottom of the casserole. If presweetened, do not add honey. If fresh, spoon on ½ cup honey. Grate lemon peel on top of peaches, then cut lemon and squeeze juice over fruit. Mix cinnamon with ¼ cup of the flour and sprinkle over fruit. Dab 2 tablespoons butter over flour.

In a separate bowl, combine the remaining flour, wheat germ, baking powder and salt.

In a small saucepan, heat the remaining honey, butter and milk until thinned. Add to flour mixture. Stir thoroughly, then mix in eggs and yolks. Pour batter over the fruit in the casserole.

Bake for 30 minutes, then place a large plate over top of the casserole and quickly invert so peaches are on top. Serve warm with cream.

REAL LEMONADE

MAKES: 1 quart
PROTEIN: none

Ice cubes
Juice of 5 lemons
3 cups boiling water
¼ cup honey

Fill a large pitcher half way with ice cubes. Squeeze in lemon juice. In a separate pan dissolve honey in boiling water. Pour honey water into the pitcher and stir. Refrigerate to chill or serve over more ice in tall glasses. Decorate with a slice of lemon or a few mint leaves.

RHUBARB WITH PINEAPPLE SAUCE

MAKES: 4 servings
PROTEIN: 1 gram per serving

2 cups canned pineapple, puréed
2 cups rhubarb, in 2-inch pieces
1 cup cranberry sauce
½ cup honey
1 teaspoon cinnamon

Preheat oven to 375°. Butter a small casserole.

Smooth cranberry sauce over the bottom and sides of the casserole. Add rhubarb pieces, honey and cinnamon, then cover with pineapple.

Bake 25 minutes or until rhubarb is tender. Serve warm.

STEWED PRUNES WITH CASHEWS

MAKES: 4 servings
PROTEIN: 8 grams per serving

> *1½ cups boxed prunes, pitted*
> *½ cup raisins*
> *½ cup cream sherry*
> *½ cup honey*
> *½ teaspoon ground cloves*
> *1 cup whipped cream*
> *1 cup cashews, chopped*

In a saucepan, cook prunes and raisins in sherry and honey for ½ hour. Add water if needed to prevent sticking. Sprinkle cloves over stewed fruit and stir. Mixture should be thick but not dry.

Cool to room temperature. Fold in whipped cream. Sprinkle generously with cashews.

STRAWBERRY PIE

MAKES: 6 servings
PROTEIN: 2 grams per serving

Crust

> *1⅔ cups graham-cracker crumbs*
> *¼ cup butter, in small pieces*
> *1 egg, beaten*

Preheat oven to 375°.

In a bowl, combine all ingredients and blend with a fork or fingertips until mixture is uniform. Turn out into an ungreased pie tin and press into an even-layered crust.

Bake for 8 minutes. Remove from oven and let cool to room temperature.

Filling

> 2 cups fresh strawberries, hulled
> 1 cup strawberry preserves, made with honey

Combine ingredients in a bowl. Spoon into baked pie crust. Refrigerate ½ hour.

Topping

> 1 cup whipped cream, beaten stiff
> ½ cup shredded coconut, unsweetened and toasted

Spoon whipped cream over pie. Sprinkle coconut over top. Serve cold.

STUFFED DATES

MAKES: 1 cup
PROTEIN: 21 grams per cup

> 1 cup dates
> 1 cup walnut halves

Remove pits from dates and replace each pit with 1 walnut half. Serve as a snack. To vary, use cream cheese instead of walnuts.

TROPICAL ORANGES

MAKES: 4 servings
PROTEIN: 2 grams per serving

> *4 large navel oranges*
> *2 bananas, sliced*
> *Juice of 1 lemon*
> *4 tablespoons candied ginger, finely chopped*
> *2 tablespoons honey*
> *¼ cup orange juice*

Peel oranges and slice into circular shapes. Place in a flat serving dish. Cover with bananas. Sprinkle bananas with lemon juice. Add layer of ginger bits.

Mix honey and orange juice in a separate cup. Pour over fruit. Cover and refrigerate overnight. Serve cold.

VI.
Vegetables

ANTIPASTO

MAKES: 4 servings
PROTEIN: 14 grams per serving

> *1 head lettuce, quartered*
> *½ cup Italian sweet peppers, pickled*
> *½ cup black olives, pitted*
> *4 slices Provolone cheese*
> *4 slices Capicolo, or other spiced ham, thinly sliced*
> *8 marinated artichoke halves*
> *½ cup pimiento strips*
> *4 anchovy fillets*
> *4 hard-boiled egg halves*
> *Oil and Vinegar Dressing (see page 176)*

On a serving platter, arrange bed of lettuce leaves. Arrange other ingredients attractively and dress with oil and vinegar.

BROCCOLI PARMESAN

MAKES: 4 servings
PROTEIN: 6 grams per serving

>   2 packages frozen broccoli or 1½ pounds fresh, steamed
>   ¼ cup butter
>   ½ cup Parmesan cheese, grated

In a bowl, mash broccoli heads with fork, removing any tough stems. Add butter and cheese. Mix thoroughly. Serve hot.

CARROT-RAISIN SALAD

MAKES: 4 servings
PROTEIN: 3 grams per serving

>   2 cups raw carrots, peeled and grated coarsely
>   ½ cup raisins
>   ½ cup walnuts, chopped
>   6 tablespoons mayonnaise
>   Pepper

In a bowl, combine all ingredients and serve cold.

CARROT SOUP

MAKES: 4 bowls
PROTEIN: 5 grams per bowl

> 2 tablespoons butter
> ¾ cup onions, chopped
> 3 cups raw carrots, peeled and grated coarsely
> 1 potato, peeled and thinly sliced
> 2 teaspoons tomato paste
> 3 cups chicken broth
> Paprika

In a large saucepan, cook onions in butter until soft. Add remaining ingredients and cook over medium heat for 30 minutes or until carrots are very soft.

Pour soup into a blender and mix for 10 seconds, or beat with an electric mixer while soup is still in saucepan.

Serve hot, garnished with a sprinkle of paprika.

CHARLOTTE'S GAZPACHO

MAKES: 6 servings
PROTEIN: 2 grams per serving

1 cup soft bread crumbs
2 tablespoons wine vinegar
3 large garlic cloves, crushed
1 teaspoon salt
4 tablespoons olive oil
1 large can peeled tomatoes
    (16 oz.) or 6 large, ripe
    tomatoes

Water (about 3 cups)
Vinegar and salt to taste
    (optional)
1 large cucumber, peeled and
    diced
2 large green peppers, diced
1 cup croutons

Combine bread crumbs, vinegar, garlic, salt, olive oil and tomatoes in a blender or food processor. Blend until very smooth. Add water and chill. You may want to add more water, vinegar or salt to taste before serving. Serve with cucumber, peppers and croutons as a garnish.

CHEF SALAD

MAKES: 4 servings
PROTEIN: 16 grams per serving

> ½ head of lettuce
> 2 tomatoes, chopped
> 1 medium onion, chopped
> 2 stalks celery, chopped
> ½ cup stuffed Spanish olives, sliced
> ½ cup cooked chicken, in julienne strips
> ½ cup cooked ham, in julienne strips
> 2 slices Swiss cheese, in julienne strips
> 2 hard-boiled eggs, sliced
> Oil and Vinegar Dressing (see page 176)

In a large salad bowl, tear the lettuce into pieces, then add all other ingredients. Toss with dressing and serve.

CHINESE ASPARAGUS SALAD

MAKES: 4 servings
PROTEIN: 2 grams per serving

> 2 pounds fresh asparagus, steamed
> ¼ cup soy sauce
> 2 teaspoons olive oil
> 2 teaspoons honey
> ¼ cup sesame seeds

Place the cooked asparagus in a flat serving dish. In a separate cup, mix remaining ingredients and pour over asparagus. Refrigerate for ½ hour before serving.

COLESLAW DELUXE

MAKES: 4 servings
PROTEIN: 4 grams per serving

> 2 cups cabbage, grated coarsely
> 1 cup raw carrots, peeled and grated coarsely
> 1 cup pineapple chunks
> ½ cup yellow raisins
> ½ cup walnuts, chopped
> ¼ cup mayonnaise
> ¼ cup sour cream
> ¼ cup honey
> Nutmeg
> Salt and pepper

Combine cabbage, carrots, pineapple, raisins and walnuts in a salad bowl.

In a separate cup, mix mayonnaise, sour cream and honey. Pour dressing over ingredients in bowl. Sprinkle with nutmeg, season, toss and serve.

CORN CHOWDER

MAKES: 6 bowls
PROTEIN: 8 grams per bowl

> ¼ cup onions, chopped
> 3 tablespoons butter
> 2 cups frozen corn
> 2 cups milk
> ½ cup powdered milk
> 2 cups potatoes, peeled and diced
> 1 cup Cream Sauce (see page 174)
> Salt and pepper
> Paprika

In a large saucepan, sauté onions in butter until soft. Add corn, milk, powdered milk and potatoes and simmer over medium heat about 15 minutes, or until potatoes are tender, but not mushy. Add cream sauce and bring just to boiling point. Season and serve hot.

CUBAN BLACK BEANS

MAKES: 4 cups
PROTEIN: 12 grams per cup

> *1½ cups black beans*
> *1 large onion, chopped*
> *1 large green pepper, chopped*
> *¼ teaspoon garlic powder*
> *6 tablespoons olive oil*
> *2 bay leaves*
> *1 tablespoon salt*
> *1 teaspoon pepper*
> *½ cup pimientos, chopped*
> *2 tablespoons vinegar*
> *2 dashes Tabasco sauce*

Cook beans in 2 quarts of water for 2 hours or until tender. Reserve liquid.

In a large saucepan, sauté onion and green pepper with garlic powder in olive oil until soft. Add beans and 2 cups of the water in which beans were cooked. Add seasonings and pimiento and simmer over low heat for ½ hour. Add more salt and pepper if needed. Serve hot or cold.

FRENCH ONION SOUP

MAKES: 4 bowls
PROTEIN: 20 grams per bowl

> *3 cups onions, thinly sliced*
> *½ cup butter*
> *3 cups beef broth*
> *½ cup Parmesan cheese, grated*
> *4 thick slices Vermont Brown Bread (see page 184)*

In a saucepan, sauté onions in butter until soft. Add broth and simmer for 20 minutes.

Place slices of brown bread in the bottom of soup bowls. Pour in soup and garnish with cheese. Serve hot.

GREEK SALAD

MAKES: 4 servings
PROTEIN: 9 grams per serving

> *½ large head Romaine lettuce*
> *1 cucumber, unpeeled and sliced*
> *2 tomatoes, cut in sections*
> *1 large onion, thinly sliced*
> *1 cup large green olives*
> *1 cup Feta cheese, cut in 1-inch chunks*
> *6 anchovy fillets*
> *Oil and Vinegar Dressing (see page 176)*

Place all ingredients in a large salad bowl. Toss with dressing just before serving.

GREEN BEAN SALAD

MAKES: 4 servings
PROTEIN: 1 gram per serving

> *1 pound fresh green beans or 2 packages frozen,*
> *steamed until tender*
> *½ cup vinegar*
> *1 cup olive oil*
> *Salt and pepper*

Place green beans in a flat serving dish. Pour in oil, vinegar and seasonings. Toss lightly. Let sit at room temperature for one hour before serving.

GREEN PEPPER SALAD

MAKES: 4 servings
PROTEIN: 1 gram per serving

> *1 cup onions, thinly sliced*
> *3 cups sweet green peppers, sliced*
> *¼ cup olive oil*
> *Salt and pepper*

In a skillet, sauté onions and peppers in olive oil until soft. Season and let cool to room temperature.

NANCY'S EGGPLANT SALAD

MAKES: 4 servings
PROTEIN: 2 grams per serving

> *4 tablespoons butter*
> *1 teaspoon garam masala* *
> *1 large eggplant, cut in cubes*
> *1 cup green beans, chopped*
> *2 tomatoes, cut in wedges*
> *2 tablespoons raisins*
> *2 tablespoons coconut, grated*

In a large skillet, melt butter and sauté garam masala until fragrant. Add eggplant and beans, cover and cook until tender. Add tomatoes, raisins and coconut and cook another 5 minutes until raisins plump up and tomatoes are heated through.

Serve warm.

* This spice is available at Indian specialty stores.

RATATOUILLE

MAKES: 8 servings
PROTEIN: 3 grams per serving

> *1 six-ounce can tomato paste*
> *5 cups ripe tomatoes, sliced*
> *1 large eggplant, sliced ¾ inch thick*
> *2 medium zucchini, sliced ½ inch thick*
> *2 cups summer squash, sliced ½ inch thick*
> *2 cups green peppers, chopped*
> *2½ cups onions, thinly sliced*
> *¾ cup or more olive oil*
> *½ cup sweet basil*
> *¼ cup rosemary*
> *2 tablespoons garlic powder*
> *1 cup fresh parsley, chopped*
> *Salt and pepper*

In a large skillet, sauté eggplant, zucchini, squash, peppers and onions in succession in olive oil.

Mix seasonings together in a small bowl.

Coat the bottom of a large soup pot with olive oil left from sautéing. Add layer of tomato paste, then layer of each vegetable in order, seasoning each layer in succession. Reserve a few eggplant slices for top.

Bring contents to a boil over medium-high heat, cover and reduce heat. Simmer for 30 minutes, occasionally bringing up some liquid to baste top of casserole.

Serve hot or cold.

RED CABBAGE SALAD

MAKES: 4 servings
PROTEIN: 1 gram per serving

> 2 cups red cabbage, shredded
> 1 cup raw carrots, peeled and grated coarsely
> 1 cup celery, chopped
> 1 cup tart apples, chopped
> ½ cup mayonnaise
> ¼ cup pineapple juice

Mix all ingredients in a salad bowl. Serve chilled.

SALAD NIÇOISE

MAKES: 6 servings
PROTEIN: 13 grams per serving

> 2 cups boiled potatoes, quartered
> 1 cup string beans, steamed
> 1 cup (2 jars) marinated artichoke hearts
> 1½ cups ripe tomatoes, quartered
> 1 cup green pepper, sliced into strips
> 6 anchovy fillets
> 1 six-ounce can tuna fish, packed in oil
> 1 cup black olives
> 3 tablespoons capers
> 2 tablespoons tarragon
> 3 hard-boiled eggs, sliced
> Oil and Vinegar Dressing (see page 176)

Line bottom of a large salad bowl with potatoes, then arrange other ingredients attractively on top of them. Flake tuna and spread around. Stud top with olives and capers. Sprinkle tarragon and garnish with egg slices. Moisten everything with dressing, but do not toss. Serve immediately.

SPINACH-ORANGE SALAD

MAKES: 4 servings
PROTEIN: 2 grams per serving

> 2 cups raw spinach, washed
> 2 oranges, peeled and sliced ½ inch thick
> 1 cup onions, thinly sliced
> Oil and Vinegar Dressing (see page 176)
> ¼ cup orange juice concentrate
> 1 tablespoon rosemary

Tear spinach into pieces, removing stems. Place in a large salad bowl with oranges and onions.

In a separate cup, mix dressing with orange juice and rosemary. Pour over contents of bowl, toss and serve.

STRING BEAN CASSEROLE

MAKES: 4 servings
PROTEIN: 14 grams per serving

> 2 cups string beans, steamed
> ½ cup onions, chopped
> 2 tablespoons whole-wheat flour
> ½ teaspoon salt
> ¾ cup yoghurt
> 2 tablespoons honey
> 1 cup crisp bacon, crumbled
> 4 slices Swiss cheese, grated coarsely
> 1 cup almonds, finely chopped

Preheat oven to 350°. Generously butter a casserole or baking dish.

Place beans and onions in casserole. Mix in flour, salt, yoghurt and honey. Add a layer of bacon and a layer of cheese. Top with almonds.

Bake 20 to 25 minutes or until cheese melts and starts to sink into casserole. Serve hot.

STUFFED CELERY

MAKES: 4 large stalks
PROTEIN: 2.5 grams per stalk

> *4 large celery stalks, washed*
> *¼ cup cottage cheese*
> *¼ cup cream cheese*
> *¼ cup fresh parsley, chopped*
> *1 teaspoon garlic or onion powder*
> *Salt and pepper*
> *Paprika*

In a small bowl, mix cheese and seasonings. Press into cavity of stalks. Garnish with paprika and serve.

TOMATO SALAD WITH BASIL

MAKES: 4 servings
PROTEIN: 5 grams per serving

> *4 cups ripe tomatoes, sliced*
> *1 cup fresh basil leaves, finely chopped*
> *¼ teaspoon garlic powder*
> *½ cup Parmesan cheese*
> *½ cup olive oil*

Place tomatoes in a flat serving dish. In a separate cup, mix remaining ingredients to form a paste.

Spread tomatoes with basil mixture and serve.

RECIPE INDEX

Note: Recipes are organized in groups according to the types of foods they emphasize. The first page listing shows where the dish is used in a menu. The second reference, in heavy type, indicates where the recipe can be found.

216

protein counter

I. ANIMAL SOURCES (complete proteins)

FOOD	SERVING SIZE	PROTEIN (GRAMS)
DAIRY PRODUCTS		
Butter	¼ lb. (½ cup)	0
Buttermilk	1 cup	9
Cheese		
Cheddar	1 oz. (1 tablespoon)	7
Cottage (creamed)	4 oz. (½ cup)	15
Cottage (uncreamed)	4 oz. (½ cup)	19
Cream	1 oz. (2 tablespoons)	2
Gouda	1 oz.	7
Meunster	1 oz.	6
Mozzarella	1 oz.	6
Parmesan	1 oz.	10
Ricotta	4 oz. (½ cup)	19
Roquefort	1 oz.	6
Swiss	1 oz.	7
Cream		
Light	½ cup	4
Heavy	½ cup	2
Sour	1 cup	9
Egg	1	6
Egg yolk	1	3
Ice milk	1 cup	9
Mayonnaise	1 tablespoon	trace
Milk		
Evaporated, undiluted	1 cup	16
Powdered, dry	1 cup	25
Skim	1 cup	9
Whole	1 cup	8
Yoghurt	1 cup	8

PROTEIN COUNTER (2)

FOOD	SERVING SIZE	PROTEIN (GRAMS)
MEAT AND POULTRY Figures are for cooked, edible portions (no bones or trimmings) unless otherwise indicated.		
Beef		
Chuck roast	4 oz.	23
Corned	4 oz.	22
Dried, chipped	4 oz.	25
Ground, lean	4 oz.	22
Round steak	4 oz.	24
Sirloin steak	4 oz.	20
Bologna	2 slices	7
Chicken	4 oz.	23
Duck	4 oz.	13
Lamb		
Chop	4 oz.	18
Leg	4 oz.	20
Stew pieces	4 oz.	18
Liver		
Beef	4 oz.	20
Chicken	4 oz.	20
Liverwurst	1 oz.	4
Pork		
Bacon, crisp	1 slice	2
Chop	4 oz.	16
Ham slice, cured	4 oz.	16
Ham, lunchmeat	2 oz.	13
Hot dog	1	7
Loin, roast	4 oz.	21
Salt	4 oz.	5
Sausage, links	4 oz.	11
Spareribs, bone in	4 oz.	9

PROTEIN COUNTER (3)

FOOD	SERVING SIZE	PROTEIN (GRAMS)
Rabbit, stew pieces	4 oz.	17
Turkey	4 oz.	23
Veal		
Cutlet	4 oz.	23
Stew pieces	4 oz.	23

SEAFOOD Figures are for cooked, edible portions unless otherwise noted.

FOOD	SERVING SIZE	PROTEIN (GRAMS)
Anchovies	1 oz.	5
Bass, pan fried	4 oz.	21
Clams, steamed	4 oz.	12
Cod, baked fillet	4 oz.	24
Crabmeat, cooked	4 oz.	14
Flounder, baked fillet	4 oz.	25
Haddock, fried fillet	4 oz.	16
Halibut, baked fillet	4 oz.	16
Herring		
fresh	4 oz.	14
kippered	4 oz.	23
Lobster, steamed	4 oz.	19
Mackerel		
fresh	4 oz.	25
smoked	4 oz.	27
Mussels, steamed	4 oz.	26
Oysters, raw	6–8 medium	8
Perch, pan fried	4 oz.	22
Pike, pan fried	4 oz.	21
Red snapper, baked fillet	4 oz.	22
Rockfish, baked fillet	4 oz.	21
Roe (Caviar)	4 oz.	28

PROTEIN COUNTER (4)

FOOD	SERVING SIZE	PROTEIN (GRAMS)
Salmon		
Canned	4 oz.	24
Smoked	4 oz.	24
Steak	4 oz.	25
Sardines, canned	1 oz.	5
Scallops, baked	4 oz.	17
Shrimp, cleaned, steamed	4 oz.	20
Trout, pan fried	4 oz.	22
Tuna, canned	4 oz.	28

II. VEGETABLE SOURCES (incomplete proteins)
NUTS AND SEEDS Except as indicated, 4 oz. nutmeats equals 1 cup.

Almonds	4 oz.	21
Brazil nuts	4 oz.	16
Cashews	4 oz.	19
Chestnuts, uncooked	4 oz.	3
Coconut, grated	2 oz. (⅝ cup)	2
Filberts	4 oz.	14
Macadamias	4 oz.	9
Peanuts, roasted	4 oz.	30
Peanut butter	⅓ cup	12
Pecans	4 oz.	10
Pignoli (pinenuts)	4 oz.	35
Sesame seeds	2 oz. (⅓ cup)	5
Sunflower seeds, hulled	2 oz. (½ cup)	13
Walnuts	4 oz.	17
Water chestnuts	4 oz.	1

PROTEIN COUNTER (5)

FOOD	SERVING SIZE	PROTEIN (GRAMS)

DRIED BEANS Figures are for uncooked beans. Beans swell dramatically as they cook, absorbing more water the longer they soak or simmer. Some estimates of total yield are given.

FOOD	SERVING SIZE	PROTEIN (GRAMS)
Black turtle beans	4 oz. (⅝ cup)	25
Black-eyed peas (Cowpeas)	4 oz.	24
Chickpeas (Garbanzos)	4 oz. (½ cup) yield—1½ cups	23
Kidney beans	4 oz. (⅜ cup) yield—2¼ cups	26
Lentils	5 oz. (⅔ cup)	35
Mung beans	4 oz.	27
Mung bean sprouts	4 oz.	4
Navy beans	4 oz. (⅔ cup) yield—1½ cups	25
Pinto beans	4 oz.	26
Split peas	8 oz. (1 cup) yield—2½ cups	27
Soybeans	3½ oz. (½ cup) yield—1½ cups	38
Soybean curd (tofu)	4 oz.	9
Soybean milk powder	4 oz.	47
Soybean sprouts	4 oz.	7
Soy sauce	¼ cup	3

PROTEIN COUNTER (6)

FOOD	SERVING SIZE	PROTEIN (GRAMS)
FLOURS AND GRAINS Figures are for uncooked portions, unless noted.		
Arrowroot powder	1 oz. (¼ cup)	2.5
Barley	4 oz. (½ cup)	10
Bran, 100%	2 oz. (1 cup)	9
Carob powder	2 oz.	2.5
Cocoa	1 oz. (¼ cup)	4.5
Corn		
flakes, ready-to-eat	1 oz. (⅔ cup)	2
grits	4 oz. (½ cup)	10
meal	5 oz. (½ cup)	11
starch	1 tablespoon	trace
Oats, rolled	3 oz. (1 cup)	16
Popcorn, popped	2 cups	3
Rice		
brown	7 oz. (1 cup) yield—4 cups	15
puffed, ready-to-eat	½ oz. (¾ cup)	1
Soy flour		
full fat	4 oz. (1 cup)	41
defatted	4 oz. (1 cup)	54
Whole wheat		
flour	4 oz. (1 cup)	15
germ	1 cup	27
shredded	1 biscuit	3
Wheatena	1 oz. (¼ cup)	4
PASTA Uncooked		
Noodles, Chow Mein, canned	4 oz.	15
Noodles, egg	2⅔ oz. (1 cup) yield—1¾ cups	7

PROTEIN COUNTER (6)

FOOD	SERVING SIZE	PROTEIN (GRAMS)
Macaroni, Buitoni		
high-protein	2 oz.	12
Spaghetti, Buitoni		
high-protein	2 oz.	12
FRUIT		
Apple	1 medium	trace
Apricot		
fresh	3 medium	1
dried	4 oz.	5
Avocado	1 large	4
Banana	1 medium	1
Blackberry, fresh/frozen	1 cup	2
Blueberry, fresh/frozen	1 cup	1
Boysenberry	1 cup	trace
Cantaloupe	½ medium	1
Cherry, fresh	1 cup	1
Cranberry		
fresh	1 cup	trace
sauce	1 cup	trace
Currant	1 cup	2
Date, dried, pitted	1 cup	4
Fig, dried	3 large	3
Grape	1 cup	1
Grapefruit	½ medium	1
Guava, fresh	1 large	1
Honeydew melon	½ medium	1
Lemon	1 medium	1
Lime	1 medium	trace
Nectarine	1 medium	trace
Orange	1 medium	2

PROTEIN COUNTER (7)

FOOD	SERVING SIZE	PROTEIN (GRAMS)
Papaya	1 medium	trace
Peach	1 medium	1
Pear	1 medium	1
Pineapple, diced	1 cup	1
Plum	4 medium	1
Prune		
dried, soft	4 oz.	2.5
stewed	1 cup	3
Pumpkin, raw	1 cup	trace
Quince	1 medium	trace
Raisin	½ cup	2
Raspberry, fresh/frozen	1 cup	trace
Rhubarb, cooked	1 cup	1
Strawberry, fresh/frozen	1 cup	trace
Tangerine	1 medium	1
Watermelon	1 slice	2
VEGETABLES		
Artichoke, globe	1 large	2
Asparagus	6 spears	1
Beans		
green/string	1 cup	1
lima	1 cup	8
Beet greens, cooked	1 cup	2
Beets, cooked	1 cup	1
Broccoli, cooked	1 cup	5
Brussels sprouts, cooked	1 cup	6
Cabbage		
raw	1 cup	1
cooked	1 cup	2
Carrots, raw/cooked	1 cup	1

PROTEIN COUNTER (8)

FOOD	SERVING SIZE	PROTEIN (GRAMS)
Cauliflower, cooked	1 cup	3
Celery	1 stalk	1
Collard greens, cooked	1 cup	5
Corn		
on cob	1 ear	3
cooked	1 cup	5
Cucumber, sliced	½ cup	trace
Dandelion greens, cooked	1 cup	5
Eggplant, cooked	1 cup	2
Escarole	½ head	1
Kale, cooked	1 cup	4
Lettuce		
Iceberg	¼ head	trace
Romaine	¼ head	1
Mushrooms, cooked	½ cup	2
Mustard greens, cooked	1 cup	3
Okra, cooked	½ cup	trace
Olives, pitted	10 medium (½ cup)	1
Onions		
cooked	1 cup	2
raw	1 cup	1
Parsley, fresh	¼ cup	trace
Peas		
fresh/frozen	1 cup	5
canned	1 cup	3
Peppers, raw, sweet	1 large	1
Pimiento, canned	1 pod	trace

PROTEIN COUNTER (9)

FOOD	SERVING SIZE	PROTEIN (GRAMS)
Potato		
boiled/baked	1 medium	2
chips	10	1
French fries	10	1
hash browns	¾ cup	4
Radishes	5	trace
Spinach		
cooked	1 cup	3
raw	1 cup	1
Squash, cooked		
summer	1 cup	1
winter	1 cup	4
Sweet potato		
baked	1 medium	2
mashed	1 cup	3
Tomato		
canned, whole	1 cup	2
paste	4 oz. (½ cup)	4
purée	1 cup	5
raw	1 medium	1
stewed	1 cup	2
Turnip	1 large	1
Turnip greens, cooked	1 cup	4
Watercress	1 cup	1
BEVERAGES		
Apple juice	1 cup	trace
Apricot juice	1 cup	1
Beer	1 cup	trace
Bouillon/broth/consommé (canned)	1 cup	5

PROTEIN COUNTER (10)

FOOD	SERVING SIZE	PROTEIN (GRAMS)
Cocoa, made with milk	1 cup	8
Cranberry juice	1 cup	trace
Eggnog	1 cup	12
Grapefruit juice	1 cup	1
Grape juice	1 cup	1
Lemon juice, fresh	½ cup	trace
Lime juice, fresh	½ cup	trace
Milk	1 cup	8
Orange juice	1 cup	2
Pineapple juice	1 cup	1
Prune juice	1 cup	1
Tomato juice	1 cup	2
Club soda	1 cup	0
Coffee, black	1 cup	trace
Colas	1 cup	0
Fruit-flavored "drink," canned/powdered	1 cup	0
Ginger ale	1 cup	0
Liquor	1 oz.	0
Powdered "breakfast drink"	1 cup	0
Powdered imitation soda	1 cup	0
Root beer	1 cup	0
Tea, plain	1 cup	trace
Wine	½ cup	trace
SWEETS		
Candy		
caramels	5	trace
fudge	2 pieces	trace
marshmallows	5	1
milk chocolate	2 oz. bar	2

PROTEIN COUNTER (11)

FOOD	SERVING SIZE	PROTEIN (GRAMS)
Commercial baked goods	impossible to calculate—most are made with refined flours and sugars, and various synthetic ingredients (see Recipes for more nutritious varieties)	
Corn syrup	2 tablespoons	0
Jam/jelly/preserves	2 tablespoons	0
Honey	2 tablespoons	trace
Maple syrup	2 tablespoons	0
Molasses	2 tablespoons	0
Sugar		
brown	1 cup	0
white	1 cup	0

INFORMATION DIRECTORY

1. Society for the Protection of the Unborn through Nutrition
   (SPUN)
   Suite 603
   17 N. Wabash
   Chicago, Illinois 60602

A national organization dedicated to the establishment of scientific standards of nutrition management in American obstetrical practice. Counsels pregnant women directly and through personnel in prenatal clinics, physicians' offices and childbirth classes. Publishes pamphlet on fundamentals of prenatal nutrition, bibliography on malnutrition and reproductive casualty, and newsletter. Provides speakers for community and professional meetings. Makes referrals to childbirth specialists knowledgeable about nutrition. Telephone: (312) 332-2334.

2. Cinema Medica
   664 N. Michigan
   Chicago, Illinois 60611

Film makers whose catalog list features nutrition, childbirth and breast-feeding subjects. "Nutrition in Pregnancy," a 30-minute, 16mm, color film, features Dr. Tom Brewer and a group of expectant parents in an informal nutrition counseling session modeled on those of the Contra Costa County toxemia prevention project. Available for rental or preview in addition to purchase. Currently in use in hospitals, clinics and other health care agencies across the country.

CHILDBIRTH EDUCATION

1. American Academy of Husband-Coached Childbirth (AAHCC)
   The Bradley Method
   P.O. Box 5224
   Sherman Oaks, California 91413

A national organization which trains and certifies teachers of the Bradley Method of childbirth education, originated by Dr. Robert A. Bradley of Denver. Maintains referral service to affiliated teachers and information service (films, reprints, tape cassettes, student workbooks) on all aspects of the physiological approach to childbearing. The Bradley Method stresses sound nutrition, progressive relaxation for labor, father participation in birth and strong consumer orientation.

2. National Association of Parents and Professionals for Safe
   Alternatives in Childbirth (NAPSAC)
   P.O. Box 267
   Marble Hill, Missouri 63764

A national organization seeking to establish medically safe, family-oriented birth programs in home as well as hospital settings. Sponsors annual national conference, publishes books and carries on public educational programs.

BIBLIOGRAPHY

Acosta-Sison, Honora, "Relation between the state of nutrition of the mother and the birth weight of the fetus." *J. Philippine Is. Med. Assoc.,* 9:174, 1929.

Agriculture Research Service, *Nutritive Value of Foods.* Home and Garden Bulletin No. 72. Washington, D.C.: U.S. Dept. of Agriculture, 1970.

American College of Obstetricians and Gynecologists, Committee on Nutrition, *Nutrition in Maternal Health Care.* Chicago, 1974.

Antonov, A. N., "Children born during the siege of Leningrad in 1942." *J. Pediatrics,* 30:250, 1947.

Brewer, T. H., "Limitations of diuretic therapy in the management of severe toxemia: the significance of hypoalbuminemia." *Amer. J. Obstet. Gynecol.,* 83:1352, 1962.

————, *Metabolic Toxemia of Late Pregnancy: A Disease of Malnutrition.* Springfield, Ill.: C. C. Thomas, 1966.

————, "Human pregnancy nutrition: an examination of traditional assumptions." *Aust. N.Z.J. Obstet. Gynaecol.,* 10:87, 1970.

————, "Human maternal-fetal nutrition." *Obstet. Gynecol.,* 40:868, 1972.

BIBLIOGRAPHY

Brewer, T. H., "Metabolic toxemia of late pregnancy in a county prenatal nutrition education project: a preliminary report." *J. Reproduct. Med.,* 13:175, 1974.

———, "Consequences of malnutrition in human pregnancy." *CIBA Review: Perinatal Medicine,* Basel, Switzerland: CIBA-Geigy, Ltd., 1975, p. 5.

———, "Role of malnutrition in preeclampsia and eclampsia." *Amer. J. Obstet. Gynecol.,* 125:281, 1976.

Burke, Bertha S., et al., "Nutrition studies during pregnancy." *Amer. J. Obstet. Gynecol.,* 46:38, 1943.

Cannon, Walter B., *The Wisdom of the Body.* New York: W. W. Norton, 1963 (reissue of 1939 edition).

Chesley, Leon, "Plasma volume and red cell volume in pregnancy." *Amer. J. Obstet. Gynecol.,* 112:440, 1972.

———, Testimony to U.S. Food and Drug Administration, Bureau of Drugs, OB-GYN Advisory Committee, Rockville, Md. July 17, 1975.

Cloeren, Stella, et al., "Hypovolemia in toxemia of pregnancy: plasma expander therapy." *Arch. Gynak.,* 215:123, 1973.

Davis, Adelle, *Let's Cook It Right.* New York: Harcourt Brace Jovanovich, 1970, p. 518.

Dieckmann, W. J., et al., "Observations on protein intake and the health of the mother and baby. I. Clinical and laboratory findings." *J. Amer. Dietet. Assoc.,* 27:1046, 1951.

Dobbing, John, "The later growth of the brain and its vulnerability." *Pediatrics,* 53:2, 1974.

Drillien, Cecil Mary, "Physical and mental handicap in the prematurely born." *J. Obstet. Gynaecol. Brit. Emp.,* 66:721, 1959.

Eastman, N. J. and E. Jackson, "Weight relationships in pregnancy." *Obstet. Gynecol. Survey,* 23:1003, 1968.

Ebbs, John H., et al., "The influence of prenatal diet on the mother and child." *J. Nutrition,* 22:515, 1941.

Ebbs, John H., et al, "The influence of improved nutrition on the infant." *Canad. Med. Assoc. J.,* 46:6, 1942.

Ewald, Ellen Buchman, *Recipes for a Small Planet.* New York: Ballantine Books, 1971.

Ferguson, J. H. and A. Keaton, "Studies of the diets of pregnant women in Mississippi. I. The ingestion of clay and laundry starch." *New Orleans Med. Surg. J.,* 102:460, 1950.

————, "II. Diet patterns." *New Orleans Med. Surg. J.,* 103:81, 1950.

Ferguson, James H., "Maternal death in the rural South." *J. Amer. Med. Assoc.,* 146:1388, 1950.

Goldbeck, Nikki and David Goldbeck, *The Supermarket Handbook: Access to Whole Foods.* New York: Harper & Row, 1973.

Gray, Mary Jane, "Regulation of sodium and total body water metabolism in pregnancy." *Amer. J. Obstet. Gynecol.,* 89:760, 1964.

Grieve, J. F. K., "Prevention of gestational failure by high protein diet." *J. Reproduct. Med.,* 13:170, 1974.

Habicht, Jean-Pierre, et al., "Relation of maternal supplementary feeding during pregnancy to birth weight and other sociobiological factors," *Nutrition and Fetal Development,* M. Winick, ed. New York: J. Wiley & Sons, 1974.

Hamlin, R. H. J., "The prevention of eclampsia and pre-eclampsia." *Lancet* 1: 64, 1952.

Hibbard, Lester, "Maternal mortality due to acute toxemia." *Obstet. Gynecol.,* 42:263, 1973.

Hodin, Jay and T. H. Brewer, "Why Mothers Must Meet the Nutritional Stress of Pregnancy," in Stewart and Stewart, eds., *Twenty-first Century Obstetrics Now!,* Vol. 2, Chapel Hill, N.C.: NAPSAC Press, 1977.

Higgins, Agnes C., "Nutritional status and the outcome of pregnancy." *J. Canad. Dietet. Assoc.,* 37:17, 1976.

234

BIBLIOGRAPHY

Howard, Peggy, "Albumin concentrate can be used for mild pre-eclampsia." *Ob.-Gyn. News,* October 1, 1974.

Hytten, F. and I. Leitch, *The Physiology of Pregnancy.* Oxford: Blackwell, 1970.

Iyengar, Leela, "Effects of dietary supplements late in pregnancy on the expectant mother and her newborn." *Ind. J. Med. Research,* 55:85, 1967.

————, "Urinary estrogen excretion in undernourished pregnant Indian women: effect of dietary supplement on urinary estrogens and birth weights of infants." *Amer. J. Obstet. Gynecol.,* 102:834, 1968.

Jelliffe, D. B. and E. F. P. Jelliffe, "The Uniqueness of Human Milk." *Amer. J. Clin. Nutri.,* 24:968–1024, 1971.

Knobloch, Hilda, et al., "Neuropsychiatric sequelae of prematurity: a longitudinal study." *J. Amer. Med. Assoc.,* 161:581, 1956.

Lappe, Frances Moore, *Diet for a Small Planet.* New York: Ballantine, 1971.

Lechtig, Aaron, et al., "Effect of moderate maternal malnutrition on the placenta." *Amer. J. Obstet. Gynecol.,* 123:191, 1975.

López-Llera, Mario, *Conducta Medica en la Fase Compensada de la Toxemia del Embarazo.* Bulletin No. 4, Temas de Toxicologia, México, D.F., Consejo Nacional de Prevención de Accidentes, Secretaria de Salubridad y Asistencia, 1975.

Lowe, Charles U., "Research in infant nutrition: the untapped well." *Am. J. Clin. Nutri.,* 25:245, 1972.

Mellanby, Edward, "Nutrition and child-bearing." *Lancet* 2:1131, 1933.

Pasamanick, B. and A. Lilienfeld, "Association of maternal and fetal factors with development of mental deficiency. I. Abnormalities in the prenatal and paranatal periods." *J. Amer. Med. Assoc.,* 159:155, 1955.

Pasamanick, B. and H. Knobloch, "Pregnancy experience and

the development of behavior disorder in children." *Amer. J. Psychiatry*, 112:613, 1956.

Phillips, M. G., "The Nutrition Knowledge of Medical Students." *J. Medical Education*, Vol. 46, Jan. 1971.

Pike, R. L. and H. A. Smiciklas, "A reappraisal of sodium restriction during pregnancy." *Internatl. J. Gynaecol. Obstet.*, 10:1, 1972.

Platt, B. S., "Experimental protein-calorie deficiency," in R. A. McCance, and E. M. Widdowson, eds.: *Calorie Deficiencies and Protein Deficiencies.* Boston: Little, Brown, 1968, pp. 237–248.

Platt, B. S. and R. J. Stewart, "Reversible and irreversible effects of protein-calorie deficiency on the central nervous system of animals and man." *World Rev. Nutri. Dietet.*, 13:43, 1971.

Prochownick, L., "Ein Versuch zum Ersatz der kunstlichen Frühgeburt" (An attempt toward the replacement of induced premature birth). *Zbl. Gynak.* 30:577, 1899.

Robinson, Margaret, "Salt in pregnancy." *Lancet*, 1:178, 1958.

Ross, Robert A., "Relation of vitamin deficiency to the toxemias of pregnancy." *South. Med. J.*, 28:120, 1935.

———, "A study of certain dietary factors of possible etiologic significance in toxemias of pregnancy." *Amer. J. Obstet. Gynecol.*, 35:426, 1938.

Schewitz, Lionel, "Hypertension and renal disease in pregnancy." *Med. Clin. N. Amer.*, 55:47, 1971.

Scrimshaw, Nevin S., et al., *Interactions of Nutrition and Infection.* Bulletin No. 57, World Health Organization, Geneva, 1968.

Shanklin, Douglas, "Making pregnancy healthy." *Medical Tribune*, May 23, 1973.

Shanklin, Douglas R. and Jay Hodin, *Maternal Nutrition and Child Health.* Springfield, Ill.: C. C. Thomas, 1979.

Sheehan, H. L. and J. B. Lynch, *Pathology of Toxaemia of Preg-*

BIBLIOGRAPHY

nancy. Edinburgh and London: Churchill Livingston, 1973.

Singer, Judith E., et al., "Relationship of weight gain during pregnancy to birth weight and infant growth and development in the first year of life." *Obstet. Gynecol.,* 31:417, 1968.

Strauss, Maurice B., "Observations on the etiology of toxemias of pregnancy." *Amer. J. Med. Sci.,* 190:811, 1935.

Tompkins, Winslow T., "The significance of nutritional deficiency in pregnancy." *Journal of the International College of Surgeons,* 4:147–153, 1941.

Toverud, Guttorm, "The influence of nutrition on the course of pregnancy." Milbank Memorial Fund Quarterly, 28:7, 1950.

United Nations Statistical Handbook, New York, 1972.

Watt, B. K. and A. L. Merrill, *Composition of Foods: Raw, Processed, Prepared.* Agriculture Handbook No. 8, U.S. Dept. Agriculture, Wash. D.C., 1963.

Wynn, M. and A. Wynn, *The Protection of Maternity and Infancy.* London: E. H. Baker & Co., 1974.

INDEX

238

A selection of books published by Penguin is listed on the following pages.

For a complete list of books available from Penguin in the United States, write to Dept. DG, Penguin Books, 299 Murray Hill Parkway, East Rutherford, New Jersey 07073.

For a complete list of books available from Penguin in Canada, write to Penguin Books Canada Limited, 2801 John Street, Markham, Ontario L3R 1B4.

Sheila Kitzinger

THE EXPERIENCE OF CHILDBIRTH
Fourth Edition

The Experience of Childbirth is written by a sociologist and ante-natal teacher—herself the mother of five children—as a complete manual of physical and emotional preparation for the expectant mother. The physiology of pregnancy, the development of the fetus, and the successive stages of labor are described in detail. Sheila Kitzinger's research and teaching focus particularly on the psychological aspects of childbearing, on the preparation of both wife and husband not only for birth but also for parenthood and marital adjustment, and on a woman's changing relationship with her own mother.

Sheila Kippley

BREAST-FEEDING AND NATURAL CHILD SPACING
The Ecology of Natural Mothering

A hundred years ago, when breast-feeding was the general practice, this book would have been unnecessary. Today, it fills an urgent need. *Breast-Feeding and Natural Child Spacing* explains how the breast-feeding mother contributes to her own psychic fulfillment and to the emotional security of her child. It also shows that breast-feeding may be an ideal means of child spacing for couples who do not use artificial contraception. Sheila Kippley tells you everything you need to know about natural mothering.

Linda Gordon

WOMAN'S BODY, WOMAN'S RIGHT
Birth Control in America

Here is a definitive history of the American woman's long struggle for the right to prevent or terminate pregnancy. Tracing the story through Theodore Roosevelt's attack on "race suicide," Margaret Sanger's pioneering crusade, the opposition of religious groups and male supremacists, and the flowering of today's women's movement, Linda Gordon shows that birth control has always been a matter of social and political acceptability rather than of medicine and technology.

Jessie Bernard

THE FUTURE OF MOTHERHOOD

Declaring that the institution of motherhood in the United States is harmful to both mothers and children, this survey looks at how American motherhood came to be the way it is, at what it is now, and at what it is likely to become. Dr. Jessie Bernard points out that the current form of motherhood was determined in Victorian England and that only recently have psychological and practical changes occurred. The many topics discussed include the mother as symbol, role severance and attrition, the working mother, psychological technologies and motherhood, and revolution via reform. Above all, *The Future of Motherhood* investigates the coming possibilities of being a mother and an *individual* simultaneously. Dr. Jessie Bernard is professor emerita of sociology at Penn State University.

John L. Hess and Karen Hess
THE TASTE OF AMERICA

American food has been drained of flavor and nourishment, crammed with additives, and disguised by fancy packaging. Our cookbooks are full of nonsense, and our finest restaurants serve frozen foods with French names at intolerable prices. Worst of all, our so-called experts encourage food snobbery and promote ignorance and error. This is an angry and a much-needed book; it is also a hopeful one, for John L. Hess and Karen Hess celebrate the richness of what used to be and tell us that we can once again enjoy good food if only we resist the forces of bad taste and bad nutrition. "A peppery, zestful jeremiad about the rape of our taste buds by industrial civilization"—Alexander Cockburn, *The Village Voice*.